Y0-EFQ-989

VISION AND LEADERSHIP

MeOtzar HoRav SERIES:
SELECTED WRITINGS OF RABBI JOSEPH B. SOLOVEITCHIK

The *Me-Otzar HoRav* series has been made possible
by a generous grant from Ruth and Irwin Shapiro.

The publication of *Vision and Leadership*
has been made possible by a grant from
Dassie and Marvin Bienenfeld
in memory of their parents
Gertrude and Morris Bienenfeld ע"ה
Minnie and Leo Usdan ע"ה.

VISION AND LEADERSHIP

Reflections on Joseph and Moses

Rabbi Joseph B. Soloveitchik

Edited by
David Shatz, Joel B. Wolowelsky, and Reuven Ziegler

Published for
TORAS HORAV FOUNDATION
by KTAV Publishing House, Inc.

VISION AND LEADERSHIP
REFLECTIONS ON JOSEPH AND MOSES
Rabbi Joseph B. Soloveitchik
Edited by David Shatz, Joel B. Wolowelsky, and Reuven Ziegler

ISBN 978-1-60280-219-3

Published for
THE TORAS HORAV FOUNDATION by
KTAV Publishing House, Inc., 930 Newark Avenue, Jersey City, NJ 07306

ME-OTZAR HORAV SERIES: SELECTED WRITINGS OF RABBI JOSEPH B. SOLOVEITCHIK

• Table of Contents •

• Preface •

Vision and Leadership is the eleventh volume of the series *MeOtzar HoRav: Selected Writings of Rabbi Joseph B. Soloveitchik*. Rabbi Soloveitchik *zt"l* (1903–1993) was one of the outstanding talmudists of the twentieth century, and one of its most creative and seminal Jewish thinkers. "The Rav," as he is widely known, brought Jewish thought and law to bear on the interpretation and assessment of the modern experience. He built bridges between Judaism and the modern world while vigorously upholding the integrity and autonomy of the Jew's faith commitment, in particular the commitment to a life governed by Halakhah, Jewish law.

For over four decades, Rabbi Soloveitchik gave the senior *shi'ur* (class in Talmud) at the Rabbi Isaac Elchanan Theological Seminary (RIETS), affiliated with Yeshiva University. Generations of rabbinical students were taught and inspired by him, among them many of the future leaders of all areas of Jewish communal life. He was the halakhic authority and spiritual leader of the Rabbinical Council of America, founded the Maimonides School in Boston, and also served as the chief rabbinic figure in that city (commuting weekly between there and New York). He contributed vitally to the dynamic resurgence of Orthodox Judaism in America.

Although many of Rabbi Soloveitchik's writings and discourses have been published over the years, much additional material remains in handwritten manuscripts and tapes. The Toras HoRav Foundation was established by family members and former students to disseminate these and other works, with the aim of enhancing both our grasp of Rabbi Soloveitchik's philosophy and our understanding of the diverse topics he addresses.

This volume presents the Rav's reflections on Joseph and Moses. We hope that by experiencing the Rav's rare blend of intellectual sweep and energizing passion, readers will find the Rav's thought an invaluable and integral part of their own spiritual quests.

David Shatz
Joel B. Wolowelsky
Reuven Ziegler

❧ *Introduction*

The present volume presents Rabbi Soloveitchik's reflections on biblical narratives and characters, beginning with the Joseph stories and the Jewish people's sojourn in Egypt and ending with the story of Moses' death on the brink of return to the Promised Land. As we encounter the Rav's analyses of the various themes and episodes, we might well repeat how he characterized his method in *Abraham's Journey*:

> Besides our understanding of the semantics of the words, their style, and the historical background, there is a great spiritual message, a *kerygma*. The Torah is not concerned exclusively with past events; it is also concerned with our thoughts, our feelings, and our commitments. . . . This is certainly true of the first book of the Bible. Human destiny is reflected in Genesis—human triumph and defeat, human greatness and smallness, the potential of what man is capable of achieving, his opportunities and even his defiance of the Master of the Universe (pp. 17-18).

Through careful exegesis of verses, illuminating analyses of character, and insightful readings of *midrashim* and classic medieval commentators, the reflections in this book seek the *kerygma* of biblical stories and an understanding of what they teach us about past and present events in the life of the Jewish people.

✱ ✱ ✱

Nearly all the material in this volume is taken from lectures Rabbi Soloveitchik delivered in the mid-1970s. The material on Genesis and Exodus was delivered at the Rav's *motzaei Shabbat* lectures in Boston; the chapter "An Old Father" includes comments made in a lecture at Lincoln Square Synagogue in New York. The chapters "Moses as Judge" and "Moses as King" were Tonya Soloveitchik Memorial Lectures in 1973 and 1969, respectively. Part of "The Golden Calf and the Roots of Idolatry" was a lecture in Boston in 1958. The last four chapters, which deal with the Book of Numbers, were lectures delivered to the Rabbinical Council of America in the years 1973–1975 (the Rav had mentioned that he was preparing a book on the unity of the Book of Numbers, and apparently he had these chapters in mind as its core). The final chapter of the present book is the second part of a lecture on *Parashat Hukkat*, the first part of which appeared in *Out of the Whirlwind* under the title "The Redemption of Death."

In preparing this volume, the editors combined material from manuscripts with material from tapes. The Rav had not readied the manuscripts for publication, so editing was required. The editors provided the headings for the chapters and subsections as well as the title of the volume.

We wish to thank various people who contributed to the production of this volume: Yitzhak Berger, Debra Berkowitz, Shalom Carmy, Nadine Gesundheit, Meira Mintz, Aaron Rakeffet-Rothkoff, and Avigdor Shinan. Noa Jeselsohn and Dov Karoll checked the sources and Rachael Gelfman Schultz compiled the index.

We extend our continued appreciation to the Toras HoRav Foundation for affording us the opportunity to further bring the Rav's Torah to a long-awaiting public. We are most grateful to Rabbi Aharon and Dr. Tovah Lichtenstein for their continued guidance during the editing process and for reviewing our work at various stages.

As the newly formed Jewish nation is poised to enter the Promised Land, its historic mission lies before it. The Rav comments,

> From the viewpoint of human reason, the redemption in Egypt should have been the only one in Jewish history. The messianic era should have commenced with the Exodus. . . . Yet we believe that at some point in time all contradictions will be resolved and that the Almighty will purge the historical order of contradictions and antithetic elements. . . . The Exodus will finally be completely realized; the eschatological era will begin; only then will the redemption from Egypt be endowed with its final meaning (pp. 221-222).

May we see that day soon.

❧ *Joseph the Dreamer*

Joseph and His Brothers

The drama of Joseph and his brothers is related in three *parashiyyot*. In *Vayeshev*, the story is one of alienation, the estrangement of brother from brother. In *Miketz*, the story is one of confrontation. In *Vayigash*, we are told about reconciliation. These phases of alienation, confrontation, and reconciliation are also reminiscent of the story of *het* and *teshuvah*, of sin and repentance.

The origin of sin is not the deed itself. Just as, regarding a tree, there is a soil out of which the fruit grows, so too with sin. What idea or emotion on the part of Joseph and the brothers was the soil out of which their alienation grew?

According to the Aggadah and the Kabbalah, as explained by Nahmanides (Gen. 24:1, s.v. *berakh*), *Kenesset Yisrael*, the Congregation of Israel, is a merger of many ideas, the synthesis of all the colors in the spectrum. Indeed, it is a combination of contradictory ideas rather than merely an assembly of individuals. The source of this concept of our community is in the kabbalistic understanding of the contradictory attributes of the Almighty, which are resolved in the manner in which He implements His will. He is the manifestation of *hesed*, kindness, possessing unlimited loving-kindness for everybody, as well as *gevurah*, might, or its parallel, *din*, justice. Unlimited justice and unlimited loving-kindness are mutually exclusive, *coincidentia oppositorum*. In the Almighty, all contradictions are resolved, and there is complete harmony. The Almighty knows how to exercise unlimited love, pity, and mercy, and at the same time to be just. A human being cannot do that.

The Kabbalah and the Aggadah interpret the conflict between Joseph and his brothers as a collision of values, of axiologies, of moral purposes. Their very personalities were incongruous; they saw things differently. The division between them was so sharp that the whole experience of brotherly love vanished. If such a clash develops among strangers, it may cause tension, which can be reflected in stiff politeness and courtesy, but not hatred. However, if this kind of conflict involves brothers, it engenders animosity and sometimes hate. Apparently, among brothers there are two alternatives, love or hate. There is no intermediate stage. That is exactly what happened between Joseph and his brothers.

In my opinion, the basic mistake of the brothers was not jealousy. Rather, it was the lack of appreciation of one of the most precious gifts that the Almighty has granted humans: the sense of unity that members of a family feel for each other, a manifold ontological experience that expresses itself in love and devotion.

Neither Joseph nor his brothers appreciated this great gift. They showed a lack of understanding of a beautiful experience—the experience which the psalmist described so beautifully: "Behold, how good and how pleasant it is for brothers to dwell together in unity" (Ps. 133:1). Or, as expressed in another psalm, "Happy is one who fears the Lord . . . happy shall you be, and it shall be well with you. Your wife shall be like a fruitful vine in the recesses of your house; your children like olive shoots around your table" (128:1–3). It is the joy and experience of being together as a family, parents and siblings. I think of this during *Yizkor*, when those who have living parents leave the synagogue, and I am filled with envy, but I also regret that many do not appreciate their parents and "how good and how pleasant it is for brothers to dwell together." Had Joseph's brothers understood this, Jewish history would have taken on different dimensions, and our historical experience would be a different one.

Gratitude is a basic virtue in Judaism, and whoever proves to be an ingrate is punished. Indeed, the punishment here was that the gift of unity was taken away from the person who failed to appreciate it. The sons of Jacob were very unhappy. They envied Joseph, for he had a multicolored coat; each one apparently thought that he would have been the happiest person if his father had given him the multicolored coat instead. They obsessed over this nonsensical thought without appreciating the real happiness of being together as twelve brothers. So they lost him. They did not appreciate each other; they did not bestow love and devotion upon each other; they were hostile to each other; there was a treasure within their reach, and they did not appreciate the treasure.

Thus was Joseph taken away from his brothers. Of course, the very moment his brothers lost him, the very moment they realized the horrible, tragic mistake they had committed, the very moment the Bedouins who took Joseph away disappeared from the horizon, they regretted their deed. Suddenly they became aware of the exalted brotherly experience.

Brotherhood involves a common past and common memories. I remember when I was seven or eight, I saved up money to buy ice cream (which was a paradisiacal treat because we were very poor) and I shared it with my brother. This is a memory that unites me with him. It did not unite me with my sisters, nor did it unite me with my youngest brother. And there are hundreds of memories like that. This common past is a tremendous bond.

The fraternal experience also includes a common future, a common destiny. This common future is more of a depth experience than a surface experience. We have to dig into the recesses of our awareness in order to discover the element of common destiny.

As Jews, we have a living memory which spans centuries and millennia. We also have an awareness of a common destiny. The past is real to us; the future is also real—as real as the past. Basically, this memory of the past together with anticipation of the future are two experiences of brothers. And since Jews are brothers, "our brethren all the house of Israel," that is what unites us: the common past and the common future.

There is also a third element in the experience of brotherliness, namely, mutual trust. When I speak of a stranger, I never know, unless he has proven his friendship to me, whether he will help me if I am ever in distress, God forbid. Will he stand with me or will he be indifferent? I am never sure. However, I am sure that whenever I face problems, whenever I am confronted by evil, my brother will come to my aid. This is also a Jewish experience, an experience that goes back very far.

Frankly, if not for this experience of brotherliness on the part of the Jewish people throughout the world, we would have vanished long ago, and the State of Israel could not have existed. If we are still a living people, it is because we know the experience of brotherliness, of giving unlimited help, of sharing in the misery and agony of other Jews. We are together in suffering and in joy. When did this feeling develop?

This fraternal experience was forged during the years of misery, when Joseph missed his brothers and they missed him. It was born in the crucible of the pain Joseph felt as a servant, as a slave, and then as a lonely viceroy. It was born in the pain of the brothers when they began to regret, and to experience remorse and penitence about, the sale of Joseph. In the crucible of loneliness, distress, and grief for a brother who was lost, the idea of *Kenesset Yisrael* was formulated.

Pragmatism and Vision

In a message replete with metaphors and similes, Jacob on his deathbed addressed his sons, singling out each one's uniqueness and distinctiveness. The characterization of the brothers had great significance, because the historical responsibilities they were charged with and the nature of the tasks assigned to them corresponded to their individual talents and abilities.

When, in the most glowing and beautiful terms, Jacob tried to project the image of his beloved son, he of course singled out Joseph's beauty, charm, and charisma. Yet in his blessing the old man was not satisfied with this portrayal, and he added two enigmatic sentences:

> They embittered him and were hostile to him, and the archers shot at him and harried him. But his bow remained in imperturbable rest, and the arms of his hands were ornamented with gold, from the hands of the mighty God of Jacob, there, the Shepherd, the Rock of Israel (Gen. 49:23–24).

In my opinion, these two verses shed light on Joseph's genuine personality. There were two main traits which may account for Joseph's vigor and distinctiveness: first, strength, and second, an ambivalence or dichotomy in his character.

Joseph's strength manifested itself in the strange ability to survive with a separate spiritual identity under circumstances and conditions that warranted complete assimilation and integration. Aristotle long ago said that man is a social animal prone to join the society in which he lives, to adopt its ways and mores and level of individual distinctiveness. Man does not want to be unique and singular; he refuses to be noticeable, to stand out and hence expose himself to loneliness and isolation, which in turn breed antagonism. In a word, man succumbs to the rule of *Gleichschaltung*, disappearance in the crowd.

Joseph did not act in consonance with this rule. The hate which he aroused in his brothers was mainly due to the fact that he stood out among them. He was distinct and different; in the pastoral, nomadic, and carefree community where he was raised, his actions were peculiar. His contemporaries could not understand when he spoke of a different economy—agriculture—and of people who did not wander from spot to spot living like parasites off the fat of the land. He envisioned people who had allegiance to the land and who displayed determination to force Mother Nature to feed its inhabitants, honest people who were ready to work, till, and irrigate. The shepherds heard in amazement this fantastic story: "For, behold, we were binding sheaves in the field, and lo, my sheaf arose and stood upright; and behold, your sheaves stood round about and bowed down to my sheaf" (Gen. 37:7). They were taken aback not so much by the fact that he saw himself as the central figure and master, but by the very story that placed himself and them within a different society, not a pastoral but an agricultural one.

They resented his strangeness and singular way of seeing things more than they resented the egocentricity they wrongly imputed to him. "They embittered him and were hostile to him" (Gen. 49:23) because he beheld visions, prophesying and preaching social change. He disturbed the primitive sense of peace that entranced the naive and gullible pastoral society. The brothers were angered by Joseph's dreams and visions. "They hated him yet more for his dreams" (Gen. 37:8). They felt that in his dreams there was a spark of truth, that the voice of God broke through those dreams. But they could not listen to them. They acted just like the aristocrats of Samaria who wanted to silence the prophet Amos.

(We note that this is the reason for choosing the prophecy of Amos as the *haftarah* for *Vayeshev*. The prophet tells us that when Amos came from Judea to Samaria to prophesy and to preach, the citizens of Samaria tried to stop and silence him. They told him to return to Judea and not to prophesy in

Samaria (7:12–13). They made a mistake, as did the brothers. It is impossible to silence a prophet who was entrusted by God to carry a divine message and deliver it to people who are afraid to listen to it. He who possesses such a message is compelled to address his fellow man under all circumstances, whether he is listened to or not, even if he injures himself thereby. It is the divine influence that moves them and does not allow them to rest at all. Jeremiah said: "The word of God was to me a reproach and a mocking all day . . . but it was in my heart as a burning fire; I was wearied to keep it in and did not prevail" (20:8–9). This is also the meaning of Amos' words (3:8), "The Lord has spoken; who will not prophesy?")

No matter how much hostility he encountered on account of his novel ideas and strange thoughts, Joseph refused to change, to act like anyone else in the pastoral society. Indeed, "His bow remained in imperturbable rest." Joseph was not impressed by the formidable opposition he encountered. He did not deny his identity, his way of life, his self-esteem and determination to be himself. He could not submerge or obliterate his distinctiveness.

The second trait of Joseph's character comes to expression in the next part of Jacob's blessing, "and the arms of his hands were ornamented with gold, from the hands of the mighty God of Jacob, there, the Shepherd, the Rock of Israel." Joseph was a very practical man. He organized the Egyptian economy and ran the whole empire; he saved the Egyptian people from the worst famine; he was the statesman par excellence. He knew how to deal with people. He understood human weakness and knew human nature. However, at the same time he was a dreamer, a visionary who beheld something beautiful, mysterious. He was fascinated by a world purged and cleansed from evil, a humanity that reached the apex of moral ascent. He dreamt not only of farming, but of stars winking to him from boundless distances.

The greatness of Joseph expressed itself in that strange merger of two mutually exclusive powers: one of logical analysis, of precision, of discriminating between fact and fancy, the power of being in contact with reality, no matter how uncomfortable; and the other of dreaming, questing, and reaching out for something which reality does not have. The multicolored garment which Joseph wore—"the arms of his hands were ornamented with gold"—symbolized the very gist of his personality: dreaming and pragmatism, clairvoyance and realism. It had many colors, and it is in that contradiction that his distinctiveness was manifest.

Of course, the Jew represents the same ambivalence. He has inherited Joseph's dual nature. On the one hand, we are very practical people; we are skeptics, very critical of things and events. We examine every phenomenon in the light of matter-of-fact logic, in terms of possibilities and probabilities. We have a down-to-earth approach, and emotions do not sweep us off our feet.

On the other hand, like Joseph, we are dreamers, prophets, visionaries beholding the whole universe, hoping and believing that, even though it is slow in coming, the great day—"*ba-yom ha-hu*"—will finally arrive. And for the sake of that wondrous day we have heroically defied the whole world and retained our identity.

The dual nature of the Jew as realist and visionary has been responsible for our survival. Like Joseph, we can dream and be seers while living in a very pragmatic, scientifically oriented world.

Joseph's Dreams

Now let us understand Joseph's dreams. Hidden desires, suppressed wishes, urges which a man is ashamed to admit, an inner life of which he is sometimes ashamed or is afraid to reveal to others—all these break through in a dream. True, Joseph wanted power; however, I believe that by stating this we oversimplify his inner life. He was motivated by love and care for his brothers.

Joseph feared two things. First, he feared the complete disintegration of the covenantal community founded by Abraham, entrusted first to Isaac and then to Jacob. Joseph did not want to verbalize this fear; he did not want to tell people that he was haunted by a fear that after Jacob's death his siblings and their many grandchildren might leave the Promised Land for parts unknown. Joseph thought that as long as Jacob was alive, the house would not disintegrate. The love and respect that everybody felt for Jacob would hold them together temporarily. But what would happen after his death? Would the names of Abraham, Isaac, and Jacob sink into oblivion; would the whole covenantal community be forgotten, dead and buried? These thoughts frightened him; they troubled him constantly like a vicious ghost.

But Joseph had another vision too, one which compounded the problem of survival. Joseph beheld another vision, the prospect of exile in Egypt. Willy-nilly, the Jews would have to pay the note that Abraham had accepted, a note which demanded four hundred years of slave labor in a strange country. They would have to live in a cruel land run by a dictatorial Pharaoh, a society that tolerated no diversity. Joseph had a feeling of doom. He was afraid of the future and what it held in store. If, he thought, the house of Jacob should fall apart and enter Egypt not as a united, well-organized community, God forbid, the house of Jacob would in no time disappear in the Egyptian melting pot. Joseph realized that in order to protect the house of Jacob, it was necessary to have unity and leadership. So he began to dream about leadership, a central authority which would take the place of Jacob and be the cohesive force that would hold all of Jacob's descendants together. He beheld the vision of a tight-knit community united at the economic and political levels.

Let us now analyze Joseph's first dream. "Behold, we are gathering sheaves in the middle of the field, *be-tokh ha-sadeh*" (Gen. 37:7). Why in the middle of the field? Basically, Joseph says, I was gathering the sheaves *with* you. We were all united. No one was at the edge, no one was less important than his more talented brother, no one was in the center. We were not divided; there was no envy, no hate, no difference between me and you. I was gathering the bundles like anyone else, but somehow my sheaf stood up. I wanted to remove it from the spot and drag it toward your sheaves, but it refused to move. Not only did my sheaf act automatically, your sheaves also acted without your consent. They stood up automatically, surrounded my sheaf, and bowed down to it. In other words, neither was I eager to be the central figure nor did you sanction the centrality of my role; however, Providence did not consult with us. I will be the happiest person if the leadership is taken away from me and turned over to someone else. The question of who will be the central figure is unimportant. We cannot all be equals and guide the destiny of an economic community. Even the most democratic country needs a president endowed with power. If Providence chose me, I will take it on.

A person dreams of facts or realities which are known to him. I should have dreamt of sheep, not of sheaves, thought Joseph. Canaan was not an agricultural country. His family had been shepherds all their lives. Had this been a simple dream, it would have operated with sheep, not with sheaves. He realized that Providence was ready to make them leave the Promised Land with its quiet and peaceful pastoral society and settle in an agricultural society. A change from pastoral to agricultural economy, like any other migration from a land with a lower economy to a land with a higher economy, may have a disastrous impact within the house of Jacob. The whole community will disappear if we should not be united. To survive, we need a leader; and if Providence has placed leadership on my shoulders, I am ready to surrender.

Then Joseph had another dream. Of course, in the covenantal community there is no separation between economy and morality, between the spiritual teacher and the so-called industrial manager. The covenant is as concerned with the meal as it is with the synagogue or the sanctuary. The person who will be the leading figure in the economic area should also be the spiritual teacher of the community in heavenly matters. Joseph apparently did not want to be just an economic czar; he dreamt of both teaching and managing. The first dream concerned only one thing, economic unity and security. Beggars cannot form a covenantal community. However, the central figure in the spiritual community must deal not only with sheaves, but with the stars in heaven, with celestial matters. Joseph thought that he possessed both qualifications.

The brothers understood Joseph's dreams very well. That is why they told him at the very beginning, *"Ha-malokh timlokh aleinu, im mashol timshol banu,* Shall you reign over us, shall you have dominion over us?" (Gen. 37:8) There is a basic difference in Hebrew between *moshel* and *melekh*. The Vilna Gaon pointed it out—not in regard to Joseph, but with regard to the verse *"Ki la-A-donai ha-melukhah u-moshel ba-goyim,* For kingship is the Lord's and He rules the nations" (Ps. 22:29). We have a *moshel* when power is imposed upon a person by brute force, when a person is compelled to accept authority. A *melekh* means one elected by the people. One cannot impose oneself upon the people as a king; one must be chosen by them. There are many kings who have no kingdoms, but there cannot be a king without kingship, the inner charisma and spiritual endowment or quality which singles out a person and elevates him above the crowd.

The Vilna Gaon says that *"Ki la-A-donai ha-melukhah"* means that God should be accepted by everybody voluntarily. But unfortunately many peoples have refused to accept God, and therefore He is *"moshel ba-goyim."* God imposes His might upon them because He is all-powerful. Our eschatological hope, our messianic vision, is that God will be accepted voluntarily by everybody.

That is exactly what the brothers told Joseph. What do you want? "*Ha-malokh timlokh aleinu*" or "*mashol timshol banu*"? If you want to rule us by brute force, all right, we shall see who is more powerful. But in the second dream, you are dreaming of *melukhah*, and we will never elect you. Joseph did not want just *memshalah*, rulership; he reached out for *malkhut*, for the prerogative of being *meshiah Hashem*, anointed by God to be the king-teacher of the people, the individual to whom the sun, the moon, and the stars bowed down. The fact that the sheaves bowed down was not good enough for Joseph; he wanted the moon and the stars.

The Torah emphasizes that the first dream was told just to the brothers, the second to his brothers and his father. There is a reason for this difference. Joseph knew that it would be possible to attain economic and political power without Jacob's consent. Jacob would not determine whether Joseph should rule over his brothers. That is why Joseph did not care to tell him anything about the dream of the sheaves. However, Joseph knew that *malkhut*, kingship, is spiritual charisma rather than a political office. It would never be given by Providence to any of Jacob's children without Jacob's consent. Providence would never interfere with the exalted tradition entrusted to Abraham. In matters of Halakhah we do not listen to any voice from heaven: "*Lo ba-shamayim hi*" (Deut. 30:12; see *Bava Metzia* 59b). Only Jacob will select the king.

Thus Joseph told Jacob of the second dream—and he expected him to exclaim enthusiastically, "How wonderful! Indeed it will happen, the way you beheld in your dream!" However, instead of endorsing the dream and sanctioning division, Jacob rebuked him. "Shall I and your mother and your brothers come to bow down in front of you?" (Gen. 37:10). Joseph's main desire suddenly was fixed: to make Jacob accept the dream.

The Beginning of Jewish History

When we read the story of the sale of Joseph, many problems come up in our minds. The whole story is sometimes so mysterious, bordering on the paradoxical, that we do not understand exactly what happens.

> He [Jacob] sent him [Joseph] out from the valley of Hebron. . . . And a certain man—*ha-ish*—found him, and behold, he was wandering in the field; and the man, the *ish*, asked him, saying, "What do you seek?" And he said, "I seek my brothers." . . . And the man said . . . "I heard them say, Let us go to Dothan." And Joseph went after his brothers to Dothan, and he found them at Dothan (Gen. 37:14–17).

In recording and reporting events, the Bible never pays attention to secondary events even though they are necessary. Thus, if we were interested only in the main event, the Torah could have said, "He sent him from the valley of Hebron and he went to Dothan, and he found them there." What made him go to Dothan instead of Shechem is completely irrelevant, and the Bible never would have recorded this event if it lacked significance. The important thing is that the result of the journey was the sale of Joseph. What does it matter whether he got lost, and a man told him that he had overheard that they had decided to move on from Shechem to Dothan, and because the man told him this, Joseph went? Who is concerned with "the man"?

In general, "*ha-ish*, the man," in the Bible, is a very strange term that has multiple meanings. The recurrence of the word *ish* in the story of the sale of Joseph is noteworthy. "And an *ish* found him, saying, What do you seek? . . . And the *ish* said to him." There is no reason to repeat that it was the *ish*; it could have said simply, "He told him, 'I heard them say, let us journey from here and go to Dothan.'"

Where else do we encounter an *ish*? When the brothers report to Jacob the events and experiences they lived through in Egypt, they say, "The *ish* who is the lord of the land spoke roughly to us" (Gen. 42:30). And Jacob himself said, "May God Almighty give you mercy before the *ish*" (43:14). And when Joseph commanded the head of his household to invite the brothers to his home, the verse reports, "And the *ish* did as Joseph ordered. . . . And they [the brothers] approached the *ish* who was appointed over Joseph's house. . . . And the *ish* brought the men into Joseph's house" (43:17, 19, 24).

Ish often means in Hebrew not just an individual but one who has no business getting involved, a stranger, one who does not belong to the whole drama, one who is outside the frame of reference. "And an *ish* found him wandering in the field." This *ish* was not involved. He is a very strange personality. In *Vayeshev* and in *Miketz*, the word *ish* is used frequently because it is the story of the most enigmatic events that somehow brought about Joseph's fall and rise.

Rashi (Gen. 37:15) says that the *ish* is the angel Gabriel and not a human being. Had he been an ordinary human being, he would not have asked Joseph, "What are you searching for?" We get the impression that the *ish* eagerly wanted Joseph to inter- rogate him; he wanted to tell Joseph where his brothers were, as if the *ish* had a tremendous interest in the events which were supposed to take place. The *ish* wanted to inform Joseph cor- rectly and precisely where they were. "And Joseph went after his brothers to Dothan, and he found them at Dothan." The impression we get from between the words is that the *ish* gave him specific instructions on how to journey to Dothan and find his brothers. He was eager that Joseph should meet his broth- ers, not for the purpose of reconciliation, but for the purpose of complete alienation.

The same is true when the brothers tell Jacob, "The *ish* who is the lord of the land spoke roughly to us, and took us for spies of the country" (Gen. 42:30). "Roughly" here is not so much in the sense of angry, hard words, but it is more that this mysterious man, this paradoxical man, treated us in a confusing manner. What motivated a stranger to accuse us of being spies? No one could understand it, not even Jacob. Our Sages say that divine inspiration was withheld from Jacob (*Avot deRabbi Natan* 30; *Yalkut Shimoni* 142); therefore he answered, "May God Almighty give you mercy before the *ish*."

The common denominator between the *ish* in Shechem and the *ish* in Egypt is that their identities and motives were mysterious. What motivated Joseph in Shechem and his brothers in Egypt to act as they did? It was the feeling of strangeness, the complete lack of understanding that arose from the encounter with the *ish*. The sale of Joseph was an illogical act; by presenting the *ish*, the Torah emphasizes that, logically, it never could have become a reality.

A strange passage in the Midrash (Gen. Rabbah 85:1) lists those who could have intervened and defended Joseph and brought Joseph back to his father. They were busy. Reuben, the Midrash says, was busy because he was concerned with repentance. He realized that the mistake he had made so many years ago involving his stepmother was now responsible for the great catastrophe of a house divided against itself. Had Reuben not committed the act of showing disrespect and protest against his father, the sale of Joseph would not have taken place. The disunity of his household started when "Reuben went and lay with Bilhah his father's concubine" (Gen. 35:22). Reuben started the rebellion unconsciously; he did not want to turn his brothers to be critical of Jacob, but he did. And this was responsible for the great tragedy that almost destroyed Jacob and his sons, as well as the covenant and all its promises. That is why Reuben was busy, engaged in penitential actions, with sackcloth and fasting.

The Midrash mentions a few other cases, and then it asks, "And the Almighty?" The Midrash gives a strange answer: "The Almighty was busy preparing the light of the Messiah." He was weaving and creating the image of the messianic king. This means that the messianic king, or the idea of redemption and all the other ideas to which *Kenesset Yisrael* later committed itself, were born on the day Joseph was sold as a slave. Jewish history began on that day.

What does it mean to say that the Almighty was busy? It means that the Almighty, with all due reverence, needed to bring about the sale of Joseph, because otherwise there would not have been a Jewish history. The idea of the specific, unique mode of existence which expresses our selection—"He Who separates between sacred and profane, between light and darkness, between Israel and the nations" (*Havdalah* prayer)—could be woven only as a result of the events which took place on that day. The Almighty had sympathy, of course, with the house of Jacob, which was about to split and enter into conflict with itself. However, if the Jews were to become a chosen people, Joseph needed to be sold into slavery. This would lead to the Jews' eventual enslavement and redemption from Egypt. Since the Almighty was determined that Jewish history should be actualized, He needed to do something very unpleasant, namely, to allow the sale of Joseph. Preventing this would have meant the complete annulment of all the covenants with Abraham, Isaac, and Jacob. There would not have been a Jewish historical experience, the experience of a community chosen by the Almighty in order to implement the purpose of creation. "He was busy preparing the light of the Messiah."

Joseph in Egypt

Joseph was sold to Ishmaelites, and then he was sold to Midianites—according to the Sages there were a few sales—and then the Midianites sold Joseph to Potiphar, who is described as *sar ha-tabbahim* (Gen. 37:36). Rashi (s.v. *ha-tabbahim*) says that this means he was the head butcher, but Nahmanides, Targum Yonatan, and most *midrashim* say that he was Pharaoh's chief executioner. You can imagine what kind of an "ethical" personality this fellow was! There were so many ways that Divine Providence could have arranged for Joseph to be introduced to Pharaoh. He could have been sold to a very decent person in Egypt, a prominent citizen who was very close to Pharaoh, and this citizen, being impressed with Joseph's wisdom, could have recommended Joseph to Pharaoh. Why did Joseph need to be sold to Midianites and Ishmaelites? They were slave traders, and even in antiquity these were the dregs of society. Why was he then sold to the chief executioner, where murder and bloodshed and injustice and cruelty were the order of the day, and then had to spend so much time in a cruel Egyptian jail? Why did God decree that the house of Jacob should be exiled to Egypt for so many years, be oppressed and tortured, enslaved and humiliated, and only "afterward shall they come out with great wealth" (Gen. 15:14)? Why was the Egyptian crucible of pain and indignity necessary?

In my opinion, God wanted the children of Israel, and particularly their representative, Joseph, to appreciate the code of Abraham. Do not forget that they were born into the house of Jacob, where Abraham's mores and moral laws prevailed. They were guided by Abraham's principles of morality and Abraham's ethics, whose basic cornerstones were mercy, charity, benevolence, kindness, appreciation, and human dignity. They had never seen evil or cruelty. They had never experienced a life guided by other principles.

There is an old idea that one begins to appreciate one's most precious treasure—freedom, health, parents, friendship—only after one loses it. The household of Jacob did not appreciate Abraham. I know it from my own childhood. Many times I could not understand what was so great about our household. I was brought up in a house of rabbis, in a scholarly home, but I used to find fault with my father, with my grandfather, and so forth. No one could convince me until I spent a number of years among gentiles, among Germans. I spent my time among the best of society in the academic community, and I saw many people who were supposed to be very ethical and moral. But I began to compare them with my grandfather or father, and I realized the difference. My confrontation with a non-Jewish society opened up a new world for me. It was as if a shining star had appeared on the horizon, as if a comet had suddenly exploded. I realized that my grandfather Reb Hayyim would have acted differently, that my father would have helped this person. In order to appreciate the good, you need to be confronted with evil. In order to appreciate traditional Jewish charity, you need to be confronted with cruelty. In order to appreciate the truthfulness and veracity which the Halakhah requires of every person, you need to view how politicians act. Colors can be identified only by comparing varying shades. The same is true regarding morality; appreciation is possible only if you are confronted with the opposite. And this is exactly what the Almighty wanted Joseph to see.

Joseph was brought up in Jacob's house. He took for granted that everyone should be charitable and truthful, that all who need should receive shelter, that a human life is precious and one should sacrifice oneself in order to save a human life. He did not appreciate the greatness of Jacob. Perhaps he was even critical of the old man; after all, he was young and imaginative, a very colorful personality, very capable. The clan could not become a great nation unless the children were ready to sacrifice. If every ethical system is just as good as the Torah, there is no need to make so many sacrifices for it. There must be something singular, something unique, something which sets the Torah apart from other codes of ethics. There is something sublime, something exalted in the Torah, but it is impossible to find from within. One must leave the house of Abraham and the house of Jacob for a while, and come to Egypt. First spend a few years with slave traders, then come into an aristocratic Egyptian home and observe the chief executioner. He was a decent person; after all, he entrusted Joseph with everything he had. But he administered Egyptian justice, which was so different from what the Halakhah requires. And then, in order to understand and appreciate the modesty of his mother and the saintliness of Leah, he needed to meet Potiphar's wife, so as to draw a comparison. And then he had to spend a couple of years in prison.

Joseph needed to experience this, for otherwise the Torah could not have said later, "Love you therefore the stranger; for you were strangers in the land of Egypt" (Deut. 10:19). The Jewish ethic—*tzedakah*, welcoming guests, truthfulness—is based upon one episode: "I am the Lord your God who has taken you out of the land of Egypt." In Egypt we learned just the opposite of what God now decrees. In Egypt we experienced what it means to be a stranger, an immigrant who speaks a foreign language and does not understand the language of the land. In Egypt we experienced what it meant to be a slave, to be steeped in poverty, to be surrounded by a selfish community that does not know the meaning of charity. The entire Jewish code is centered around our experience in Egypt, and that is why we became a great nation in the crucible of evil and cruelty, of injustice, tyranny, and selfishness.

Joseph maintained his loyalty to Jacob's tradition even though he had not been happy in Jacob's house, even though his brothers had sold him into slavery. Usually, when a child is bitter against his brothers, against his own kin, his first reaction is to abandon the mores, habits, and codes by which his kin abide. This is a form of protest—showing disregard for everything for which one's family stands. However, Joseph remained loyal to Jacob's traditions. "It is my mouth that speaks to you" (Gen. 45:12), he later said. Rashi explains (s.v. *ve-hinnei*): I speak the same tongue as you. He was away for a long time. He was taken away at the age of seventeen and was thirty years old when he was introduced to Pharaoh. Then there were seven years of abundance and two more years of famine. He was thirty-nine years old when he disclosed his identity to his brothers. One can forget a lot in twenty-two years. And yet, "It is my mouth that speaks to you," "I am Joseph your brother" (45:4), I am still your brother after so many years, loyal to what I learned in Jacob's home.

Pharaoh's Dreams

"*Va-yehi mi-ketz*, it came to pass at the end of two full years that Pharaoh dreamt" (Gen. 41:1). The term *ketz* occurs quite often in the Bible, and it always has the meaning of the end, as in "*Ketz kol basar*, The end of all flesh is come before Me" (Gen. 6:13) and "*Mi-ketz*, at the end of seven years you will declare *shemittah*" (Deut. 15:1).

Ketz in the talmudic and midrashic literature refers to the messianic redemption. Of course, the semantic meaning of both *ketz* and *sof* is the same: it is the end of the exile and suffering. The reason for adopting *ketz* and not *sof* as the synonym of redemption is quite obvious. *Sof* is related to all acts of termination. If it rains and suddenly stops, I may say "*sof ha-geshem*" but not "*ketz ha-geshem*." *Ketz* usually denotes the end of a continuous process of development. Wherever there is a promise to be fulfilled, or a historical experience to be consummated, the term *ketz* is the appropriate one. God promised that at some point in history the Jewish people will be redeemed. We know not when; however, the Almighty does. The time of redemption is the end of a long cathartic process. The maturation of this process is called *ketz*.

The history of Joseph is not an arbitrary sequence of coincidences. Joseph's life story represents a strict evolutionary process which shaped his career and gave him the opportunity to actualize his versatile talents. He had to spend many years in bondage. Every event had significance, as each day, week, and month contributed to the emergence of this great biblical figure. That is the reason for mentioning that it was exactly *mi-ketz* the two-year period, precise as to the day and hour. Each minute counted. When the clock struck, Joseph was ready to occupy the position of vizier of Egypt. His talent for leadership had matured. On that day, two years later, Joseph was ready. This is "*Va-yehi mi-ketz shenatayim yamim*," at the completion of two years of days. The verse emphasizes that Joseph's stay in

Egypt was predestined and planned to the minute by the Almighty.

The same will be true about the messianic redemption. We believe that it will happen at the very moment *Kenesset Yisrael* is ready. The Jewish people need to mature, to purge themselves of many bad habits and destructive emotions, of envy and pride and vanity and so forth. It is a process of *teshuvah*. But the very moment this process of *teshuvah* comes to fruition, the redemption will be immediately translated into reality.

Hazal, our sages, interpret the above verse to mean that the two years that had elapsed dated from when Joseph interpreted the dream of the butler. He had to stay two more years in prison. He was already a visionary and a dream interpreter. He had interpreted the dream of the butler and the butler was released. The butler could have approached Pharaoh and said there is a dream interpreter in jail, and Pharaoh would have freed him. But Joseph was not ready for leadership. He needed to spend two more years in preparation. When those two years passed, he was ready, mature, equipped with the qualities necessary to serve as viceroy of Egypt.

When that process had been completed, the Torah tells us, "Pharaoh dreams, *holem*" (41:1). The present tense is out of context here. The Torah should have written, "Pharaoh dreamt"—*halam* instead of *holem*. Ibn Ezra (Gen. 41:1, *U-phar'oh*) noticed this difficulty. He said that the form *Phar'oh holem* is identical with the form *Phar'oh hayah holem*. In other words, the verse tells us not about a dream that Pharaoh dreamt, but about Pharaoh as an individual. Pharaoh had turned into a dreamer, one who dreamt continually. This change in Pharaoh occurred exactly when Joseph was about to be elevated to power and glory. Suddenly a change came over Pharaoh; a hard-boiled, tough realist began to behold visions and to dream.

Pharaoh would have been upset by his dreams even if this metamorphosis had not taken place, but then he would not have chosen Joseph as the manager in charge of Egypt's economy. He would have appointed someone else, and Joseph's whole mission of bringing his father to Egypt would have failed. In order to accept Joseph's interpretation and give it preference over other interpretations offered by the wise men of Egypt, Pharaoh himself had to be a dreamer, a visionary, a man with sweep and deep insight who immediately recognized the intellectual-visionary genius in Joseph. He preferred Joseph's interpretation to others not on objective grounds but on purely subjective ones. He fell in love with Joseph because the latter struck an inner chord in Pharaoh's heart. Dreamer met dreamer. Visionary met visionary. When Providence was ready to elevate Joseph to the pinnacle of power, thus realizing his dream, the king of Egypt, Pharaoh, had to undergo a change of personality. He had gotten into the habit of dreaming, and he recognized Joseph as a man who was God-inspired, a charismatic, magnetic, and fascinating personality.

Joseph counseled Pharaoh to appoint a person who was *hakham* and *navon*, wise and insightful, and Pharaoh made an instantaneous decision that Joseph met those requirements. *Hokhmah* is what Aristotle called intuitive thinking, the primordial stage at which one does not know the answer but is instinctively guided by some mysterious light, a vision which tells him how to solve the problem. *Hokhmah* is a dream, a vision, a breakthrough of an inspired mind. Where there is *hokhmah*, there is imagination, sweep, and depth. There are feelings which will later be translated into concepts. The *navon* does the translating; he takes a vision and transforms it into a plan, an idea, and then transposes the thought or the blueprint into a reality.

As we have said, Joseph was a synthesis of two *prima facie* contradictory attitudes; inspiration and precision, fantasy and practicality, vision and a distinct awareness of an unalterable reality, poetic sweep and scientific accuracy. Pharaoh identified the unique personality of Joseph and elevated him to the highest office in Egypt. This explains also the generosity and hospitality of Pharaoh toward Jacob and his children. He was fascinated by Joseph. He felt that these foreigners were committed to something mysterious and precious. He, the dreamer emperor, wanted to share in that something.

Pharaoh said, "In my dream, behold, I stood upon (*al*) the bank of the river" (41:17). The preposition *al* has the connotation of nearness, proximity. For example, the curtain in the Tabernacle was *al* the ark (Ex. 40:3); however, it did not cover it—it separated the Sanctuary from the Holy of Holies. However, there is another meaning to *al*. *Omed al* is a biblical idiom, as in "*Ve-hinei Hashem nitzav alav*" (Gen. 28:13); Rashi (ibid., s.v. *alav*) explains that this means God was watching over him. It is not only a description of scenery or contiguity, but a description of a special relationship.

When Pharaoh saw himself "*omed al ha-ye'or*" it meant that he saw himself as the master of the river. The prophet Ezekiel says about Pharaoh, "Mine is the river, I made it" (Ez. 29:9). The Nile in Egypt is not just a river; it is the very essence of Egypt. The economy of Egypt depended on it in antiquity, and it still does. The Torah speaks of this unique factor which is responsible for abundance or famine. "For the land where you go to possess, it is not as the land of Egypt . . . where you sowed your seed and watered it with your foot as a garden of vegetables" (Deut. 11:10). The Torah is alluding to the peculiar situation in Egypt, where the local rain is not a factor. Life depends upon the Nile. Rashi says, "No other river is called 'the River' except the Nile, because the whole country consists of artificially constructed canals, and the Nile flows into them and fills them with water, since rain does not fall regularly in Egypt as in other lands" (Gen. 41:1, s.v. *va-yehi*). The river is nothing else but a symbolic substitute for Egypt's civilization.

Pharaoh saw himself "*omed al ha-ye'or*," concerned with the destiny of Egypt as a land and as a people. Every dreamer dreams about himself. Pharaoh wanted to make Egypt great, strong, and prestigious. All thoughts, hopes, and expectations are consecrated to the land whose image was identical with his. While he was thinking hard about Egypt, suddenly he saw a vision of seven cows "of pleasant appearance and fat of flesh." The butcher is not interested in whether the cow is good-looking or not; he is interested only in whether it is healthy, husky, and fat. However, Egyptian civilization wanted not only material prosperity but pleasantness. That is true of our modern civilization as well. We want to be economically sound and prosperous, to have security as far as the future is concerned, but modern man also has a very well developed sense of aesthetics and beauty. Aesthetics has become an ethic unto itself.

Pharaoh saw these beautiful cows devoured. The civilization of Egypt, in his vision, could produce wealth, plenty, pleasantness, beauty, prosperity, and security, but it also had within it satanic elements that wanted to destroy every institution to which the same Nile gave birth. Civilization, no matter how successful it is in its attempt to ease man's burden, is also capable of destroying him and everything for which he stands. The curse imposed upon Adam by the Almighty—that the environment will display hostility toward man—is a reality. It will yield its produce to man and yet conspire to destroy him.

Outwardly, the environment appears to be cooperative. Clandestinely it is out to defeat man, to trample upon him. Man pays the toll of the road. Each discovery to the advantage of man makes the life of man more precarious than before. Medicine has advanced greatly, yet sickness is in a race with it. Such phenomena as pollution of the environment increase the occurrence of degenerative diseases, such as malignancy due to the artificial addenda to our diet, or to the poisoned atmosphere. The possibility of destroying life on our globe in a few seconds, the increase in the number of mental patients, the boredom and constant fear experienced by man—what are they if not the seven other cows which came out of the river, the place wherefrom emerged the seven cows of pleasant appearance? The environment hates man who is out to conquer nature. It is forced by man to bow to his will. However, now and then, when man is not alert, the captive environment avenges itself on man.

Man builds, because by nature he is a maker and creator. Man destroys because man is a devil. From the river—the source of civilization, abundance and prosperity—emerge beautiful creatures and also the ugly cows, the satanic forces whose task it is to swallow the cows which are pleasant and beautiful to the sight. The blessings of the human civilizing experience may be completed by the demonic forces which man the genius sets free. Some philosophers have questioned whether the dream is worthwhile. Perhaps it would be more beneficial to man to inactivate rather than accelerate the process. Pharaoh was troubled in the morning, but his advisers did not comprehend his dilemma. They did not grasp that the dream cast doubt upon the whole civilizing enterprise.

Joseph not only interpreted the dream, but advised Pharaoh on how to protect the country from a famine, from the disaster which the seven cows represented. He realized that Pharaoh was interested in knowing the answer to the question of whether man should continue to civilize his life and let his technological genius advance without any control or instead should stop the advance right here and now.

Joseph's answer was as follows: Of course, man's conquest of nature brings him not only blessings but distress as well. The beautiful cows and the fine ears are always accompanied by ugly and bad ones. Man should take the risk. He was told by the Almighty to "conquer the earth" (Gen. 1:28). However, there is a limit to the civilizing gesture. Man should be creative and not fear the opposition and hostility of the milieu as long as he knows how to handle the blessings of civilization, as long as he does not get intoxicated with his accomplishments, as long he is guided by a wise and moral policy, as long as he does not reach out for infinity, for vastness and unlimited control, as long as he knows how to behave during the seven years of prosperity—to

[handwritten margin notes: "Out of 'Source of life'", "Pandora's Box", "Prometheus", "which are precisely his dispositions!"]

enjoy modestly, to produce humbly, to observe the law of happiness and success, to comply with the moral law pertaining to prosperity, a law which teaches him to share what he has with those who do not have.

Jews have succeeded in passing the test of poverty. I remember my childhood years. I walked around almost in rags. I still remember that when I was seven or eight years old, my friends in the *heder* would poke fun at me because my pants were torn. I came home crying. My mother promised me that in honor of Passover she would buy me a new suit. I remember that on *Rosh Hodesh Nisan* she called me in and said: Sorry, we don't have the money for your suit. We were not poorer than others. But we all passed the test of poverty. Poor Jews remained loyal.

However, we must also be able to pass the test of years of abundance and opulence. The manner in which we enjoy God's blessing, the seven good years, determines how we will manage to survive the seven lean years. If one is wise and lives in accordance with the morality of the plentiful in times of abundance, if one does not cross the boundaries of moderation and measure; if one does not surrender to irresponsible and boundless hedonism—then the onslaught by the seven thin-fleshed ugly cows will be a limited one, and man can manage to survive and pursue a good, knowledgeable, civilized life. However, if man fails during the seven good years of success, if he remembers only the dream of the seven good and happy years, if he exploits nature and reaches out for a voluptuous life, if he remains insensitive to the ethical norm and tries during good times to empty the cup of pleasure to its last drop—then the seven ugly cows will attack him ruthlessly and mercilessly. A cow is not a carnivorous animal; it is herbivorous. Yet suddenly the seven bad cows became cannibals, like predatory animals, because society did not know how to behave during the seven prosperous years. The capacity of an excited, persecuted, and abused crowd to commit cruelty and to take vengeance is unlimited.

That is what Joseph told Pharaoh: Your dream reflects human destiny. Conquest quite often ends in humiliation, prosperity in famine, happiness in distress. Man is indeed a creator; however, he is a destroyer as well. He moves fast, but he pays an enormous toll on his journey. The seven good cows are always followed by seven bad ones. Whatever is accomplished by the good is annihilated by the bad. This tragic dialectic is a part of human destiny. However, there is a way to avoid the distress and disaster which will be caused by the seven cows, and that is the intelligent handling of human success. Of course, you can, if you decide to ignore my interpretation, enjoy the seven years of abundance with a careless attitude—not anticipating trouble and not preparing yourself for disaster. Pharaoh and the aristocracy would be provided with nourishment, but the crowd may be nonchalantly left to starve. If this is the way you are planning to meet the future, then you may expect the worst—destruction and revolution. However, if you decide to meet the famine intelligently and feed the people, if you accumulate lots of food for people to survive times of need and distress but without profiteering or speculation, then the damage which the seven cows inflict will be very limited. On the contrary, the onslaught of the satanic forces upon civilization will, instead of annihilating, strengthen the constructive elements in our civilization. Whether the hostile demon abiding in our midst will succeed in destroying Egypt depends upon our action.

Pharaoh apparently understood Joseph. He said to his servants, "Is there another one like this, a man in whom the spirit of God dwells?" (Gen. 41:38). He then put Joseph's plan into effect.

✒ *Joseph the Ruler*

The Brothers Go to Egypt

When Jacob saw that there was food, *shever*, in Egypt, he said to his sons: Why do you look at one another? Behold, I have heard that there is food in Egypt; go down and obtain food for us there that we may live and not die (Gen. 42:1–2).

How did the noun *shever*, food, develop out of the verb *shavar*, to break? The common denominator in both is that food breaks hunger and thirst. We use the noun *shever* whenever we speak of basic food indispensable for the sustenance of the body, not of delicacies or large quantities of food. Only the basic foods and the smallest rations are called *shever*. Accordingly, the meaning of *shever* is "food rations" rather than simply "food." Jacob saw that there were food rations to be had in Egypt.

Joseph had introduced a rationing system. He sold food retail, in small quantities indispensable for the survival of each family or individual. Each head of a family had to appear before Joseph or his subordinate to be cross-examined. Hoarding was forbidden. Buying for speculation was made impossible. Each person was allowed to carry away one loaded animal. Delicacies were not sold.

Egypt had instituted a system typical of our Jewish philosophy and ethics. We read regarding the manna, "Gather of it every man according to his eating, an *omer* per head, according to the number of you shall you take it" (Ex. 16:16). Hoarding food while there are people who do not have anything is a sin. It reflects an egotistical, loveless being. In times of curses, famine, and trouble, people must share with each other whatever they possess. This is the foundation of the moral code of economics.

"Jacob saw"—what did he see? "Jacob heard" would have been more appropriate. The term "*Va-yar*, he saw" usually applies to discovering something surprising, confirming a guess or a suspicion. "*Va-yar*, he [Moses] saw there was no one there" (Ex. 2:12); "*Va-yar*, he [Jacob] saw the wagons" (Gen. 45:27). It also is related to the end of an exploring process, when one finally arrives at his destination. "*Va-yar*, he [Abraham] saw the place from afar" (Gen. 22:4). The verb is not employed when one wants to say he has learned or been informed about something.

Rashi noticed this difficulty and therefore concluded that the usage of the verb *va-yar* alludes to some kind of visionary activity, not just to seeing in the sense of being apprised. "How did he see? Did he not merely hear, as it is written [in the next verse], 'I have heard'? Rather, he saw in a holy dim vision that there was hope for him in Egypt. It was not, however, an actual prophetic vision to apprise him that the vision referred to Joseph [as still alive]."

In other words: Jacob was amazed to see that the method of distribution of the food by the Egyptian government, the adoption of the rationing system in order to avoid inflationary prices, speculation, and hoarding, reflected Abraham's economic morality, which dictates that the powerful and rich should not profit from the misery of the poor. But how was it possible for pagan Egypt, Jacob thought, to act in the spirit of Abraham? How did it display such fine moral sensitivity?

Something else baffled Jacob. There was a famine not only in Egypt but in all the Mideastern states. The adjacent countries were also suffering from the hunger. Had Egypt been guided by the pagan morality, it would have refused to sell food to other countries. Since the sale of grain to foreigners caused a reduction of the rations for the Egyptians, the latter had less for their own use on account of the benevolent policy to feed the starving all over the Middle East. Jacob simply could not grasp what made Egypt act so charitably in the spirit of Abraham. He said, "There is *shever* in Egypt," there are food rations to be had there—in other words, there is an equitable system of distribution. They sell food to foreigners. Therefore, go down and buy food rations which will just suffice to sustain our lives.

Why did the sons postpone the trip? Apparently, some indefinable fear prevented them from journeying to Egypt. Their sin, though twenty years old, began to trouble their minds and their consciences. The word "Egypt" aroused in them frightening guilt feelings, a sense of ugliness and self-hate. The criminal quite often has no courage to visit the place of his crime. The image of the slain person haunts the slayer. They dreaded to travel the same route that Joseph had traveled. They could not erase Joseph's image from their memories. It hovered steadily before them. It tortured them. They were pursued by his image! Of course, such a state of mind was the beginning of true repentance.

The Almighty had been waiting for them to experience this kind of fear, grisly guilt, and ruthless self-condemnation. The trip to Egypt accomplished it. Within this perspective, we will have to understand Joseph's performance, which *prima facie* reflected cruelty and vindictiveness. Why did he tease them? The answer is simple. Joseph tested them to see whether or not they had changed, whether or not they had reformed themselves, whether they had purged themselves of all their disjunctive and negative emotions (such as envy, ruthlessness, cruelty, egotism, and the lack of a sense of sharing and unity) which had led to the tragedy of selling a brother into slavery.

There is a need to travel into darkness! ~ Socrates — the forest

Joseph knew very well that the Egyptian exile, which would precipitate the birth and growth of a great nation, could not commence as long as the awareness of the common destiny and the feeling of oneness had not burgeoned. People who are capable of selling a brother into slavery because they envy him for the preferential treatment he receives from his father are not qualified to become a great nation. Hence, their sojourn in Egypt would be wasted, and the whole covenant with Abraham would prove to be null and void.

If this had been the case, Joseph would not have disclosed his identity and he would not have rejoined the household of Jacob, since the latter was divided against itself and did not differ from any other household. There would have been no covenant, no unique way of life; his hopes and his visions would have been extinguished. Joseph was not eager to be part of a clan that lived according to the rules of the jungle. Hence, had not they demonstrated their readiness to sacrifice for Benjamin, had not Judah defended Benjamin, had he not arrogantly accused Joseph of duplicity, had he not offered his life for that of Benjamin, had he not shown so much concern for Jacob's well-being (a thing the brothers had not cared for previously)— Joseph would have never revealed his identity to them and they would have been treated in accordance with Egyptian law. Joseph's reconciliation with his brothers was dependent upon the outcome of the controversy between him and Judah. Joseph became convinced that a basic metamorphosis had occurred. He decided that they were finally worthy of being the fashioners of *Kenesset Yisrael*.

The genuine mission did not consist in buying food; the real mission was to renew the brotherhood, to bring about the great reconciliation between an alienated brother and themselves. The departure for Egypt was meant to reunite all twelve brothers in order that their brotherly bond be transformed, in the course of a long sojourn, into a great union.

Why did the Torah use the expression "And the brothers of Joseph, ten of them, went to Egypt to buy grain" (Gen. 42:3)? It could simply have said, "And they went to Egypt." Instead, the verse states, "And the *brothers of Joseph*, ten, went to Egypt." The language is very strange.

They were now the brothers of Joseph. They remembered him and they had a very faint hope that perhaps in Egypt they would find their lost brother. They themselves had sold him, but now they were searching for him, because they had changed their attitude. The very instant they lost him, they began to appreciate him, so now they went like brothers with the intention of searching for Joseph. Of course, they were the brothers of Joseph even prior to the tragedy, but then they were only biologically his brothers, sharing just a common genetic code. Now, however, they began to experience brotherliness, and they were attached to Joseph experientially, not only biologically. This is the import of the phrase "the brothers of Joseph."

What is the significance of the verse highlighting the number ten? There is no need to tell us the number; it is obvious that there were twelve sons, but Benjamin and Joseph were not with them, so they were ten.

The significance of the number ten here is to be found in the verse "And it came to pass, when Israel lived in that land, that Reuben went and lay with Bilhah his father's concubine; and Israel heard it. Now the sons of Jacob were twelve" (Gen. 35:22). We learn from here that only twelve may comprise *Kenesset Yisrael*. Eleven could not do the job, and ten certainly not. All twelve tribes together must merge to create *Kenesset Yisrael*, that strange community with which the Almighty has concluded a covenant. Only twelve could build the house of Israel. *Kenesset Yisrael* is a merger of twelve ideas; they could not have been endowed with any charisma if even one brother were missing.

They went as ten, but they needed to find Joseph, because without Joseph there would be no *Kenesset Yisrael*. Jewish history would have not commenced if Joseph had not been found or if he had not identified himself as their brother. The reconciliation of Joseph with the brothers brought about *Kenesset Yisrael*.

That is why Joseph demanded that Benjamin come to Egypt. It was not only because he wanted to see his brother, who had the same mother. He knew that either all twelve brothers would participate in the formation of a *Kenesset Yisrael* or no *Kenesset Yisrael* would emerge. He wanted Benjamin in order to have the twelve tribes in one place.

That is what Jacob expressed on his deathbed. "Gather yourselves together that I may tell you what will happen to you at the end of days" (Gen. 49:1), meaning what historical destiny has been assigned to you. *Kenesset Yisrael* can come into existence provided all twelve tribes join together. These twelve people had different and singular personalities, yet all twelve had to unite and form a community, resolving their contradictions on a higher level, combining ideas which appear to be contradictory and mutually exclusive, into a community representing the great ideas reflected by the twelve tribes.

Providence looked upon the arrival of the ten brothers in Egypt as the prologue to Jewish history, as the first act of historical realization. The Torah calls them *"benei Yisrael"* (Gen. 42:5), the children of the great destiny, of the community that will defeat all antagonists. However, the brothers looked upon themselves as ordinary people who had come to purchase food like all other people who came to Egypt.

Joseph Meets His Brothers

> And Joseph saw his brothers, and he recognized them; but he made himself a stranger to them and spoke harshly to them. He said to them, "From where do you come?" And they said: "From the land of Canaan to buy food." And Joseph recognized his brothers, and they did

not recognize him. And Joseph remembered the dreams he had dreamt about them (Gen. 42:7–9).

Of course, the repetition of the fact that Joseph recognized his brothers is baffling. Some commentators suggested that the second verse should be translated as: Even though he recognized them, they did not recognize him. To explain their subsequent conversation, Ibn Ezra interpreted the verse to mean that at the outset Joseph identified them collectively, but later he recognized each one individually. Rashi there quotes a midrash: "When they were at his mercy, he treated them like brothers and felt sympathy for them, even though they had not treated him as a brother when he had fallen into their hands."

I would suggest a slightly different interpretation. These verses tell us about two identifications. The first identification was based on past experiences: the same people, the same characters, the same excitability, the same quick tempers, the same ruthless natures, and so on. Consequently, the memories of past years—all the pain, all the chicanery, all the beatings, and all the abuse he had taken—were awakened. Willy-nilly, his wrath was kindled. He disguised himself as a stranger and treated them harshly because he felt estranged from them.

The Torah continues to tell us that he recognized them later as brothers. Watching their faces and studying their countenances, he discovered a change. Levi and Simeon's faces had softened; they did not reflect ferocity and hardness. There was a different glimpse in their eyes; the steely gray eyes had turned blue, dreamy. Judah's face had matured; there was firmness and determination in his features. They all looked as if they were suffering from a depressive mood, as if they lacked inner peace, as if some grisly fear haunted them. In a word, they had come here with a contrite heart and humble, repenting spirit, but they did not recognize the kindness and graciousness that radiated from Joseph's face.

Suddenly, Joseph realized that the ten people who stood before him were not the same people who had sold him into slavery. His ire subsided. He understood that this revolutionary change in them was for the time being invisible, hidden. Quite often, the sinner does not know of the change that is transpiring in the inner chambers of his personality. The change must be objectified and externalized. There is a need for a catalyst to bring the change to his attention, to fashion from the amorphous and mysterious a new personality. The best catalyst is suffering and opposition. Joseph decided to frighten and confuse them in order that they themselves should become aware of their changed identity. At the first meeting, when he addressed the harsh words to them, he intended to punish them for their past crime. However, later he realized that he must not punish them for a sin committed by others. All he had to do was to inform them of the metamorphosis that had occurred within them; and this was to be accomplished by making things difficult, by testing their commitment to each other. Joseph knew that a reconciliation would take place, and hence *Kenesset Yisrael* would emerge. The Egyptian exile had commenced. He was the first one, they had come next, and finally Jacob would come. The divine decree was coming true.

Joseph recalled his dreams, which had been centered not about him but about the *Kenesset Yisrael* that would be formed out of the descendants of the brothers. Why does the Torah say that he recalled the dreams? Is it possible to forget such critical dreams that motivated the brothers to sell him into slavery? Certainly not! The answer is quite simple. He had lost faith in the dreams. He did not think that they would ever come true. He did not believe that he would ever meet his brothers again. How could *Kenesset Yisrael*, about which he dreamt day and night, be formed by eleven brothers while the twelfth brother was somewhere in slavery? But now he suddenly realized that the dreams might nevertheless be consummated. What was needed was to shock them out of the routine and monotony of a shepherd's life.

However, there was another key point concerning his dreams. The very moment the brothers bowed to him, Joseph was preoccupied with one thought: how to make Jacob come to Egypt and prostrate himself before the viceroy without knowing the viceroy's identity. He knew that Jacob would never separate himself from Benjamin; Benjamin would pull the old man to Egypt. Once Jacob came to Egypt, he would certainly observe protocol and bow down to Joseph the way the brothers did. If Jacob should do so, the second dream would be fulfilled and kingship would belong to him. There was only one way to achieve it.

There is something strange and enigmatic about Joseph's meetings with his brothers. Ten people come to Joseph and ask to buy food; they have the money and are willing to pay what-ever is necessary. Joseph says, No! You do not want food; food is just a pretext. You are professional spies. They say that it is not true, so Joseph puts up a condition: they will prove that they are sincere if they bring Benjamin. He sends them back to Canaan, arresting one of them, and gives strict instructions that without Benjamin they should not return to Egypt, even for food.

Imagine: the viceroy "without whom no man shall lift up his hand or foot" (41:44) publicly accused the brothers of spying for an enemy state and plotting to destroy Egypt. Time passed, and they came back. But instead of asking them a simple question, Is Benjamin here or not?, he organized a reception for them, as if he and they had been friends for years. Not only that; he gave them an exchange of gifts, an exchange of statements of devotion and love. And when Benjamin was introduced, Joseph says, "May God bestow His *hen*"—His love, sympathy, and compas-sion—"upon you, my son" (43:29).

It sounds crazy, plainly absurd. Earlier he had accused all ten of them of being spies for an enemy country. Now, not only does he tender a reception for them, he drinks with them and gets drunk with them! The explanation for this strange behavior is: "For these *anashim* shall dine with me at noon" (43:6). They are mysterious *anashim,* Joseph tells the majordomo in whom he confides. They are strangers; I do not know them, and that is why I act in a manner which seems absurd, ridiculous, and illogical. In a sense, Joseph could not control himself. "And they drank and were intoxicated with him" (43:34). When Joseph received the brothers the second time, he could not help himself.

The first time he met them, Joseph did not know how to act, whether to receive them as brothers and forget what they had done to him, or, on the contrary, to punish them because they deserved it. Joseph was wavering, and when he sent them back to Canaan with a demand for Benjamin, he did so also to gain time. In the interim, he might perhaps find a solution to the moral problem which confronted his conscience.

The Torah tells us that when Joseph saw his brothers, "*va-yizkor* the dreams he had dreamt about them" (42:7–9). *Va-yizkor* should not be understood in the sense of remembering, but in the sense of expecting: "*Zakhor et yom ha-Shabbat*" (Ex. 20:8) means "Be prepared for the day of the Sabbath," anticipate the Sabbath. Joseph had expected for many years that such a confrontation would take place. The question was how to act during this confrontation.

But now, when the brothers came the second time, he could not help himself and he had to treat them as brothers. They drank and they were intoxicated—intoxicated in the sense of being confused. The first time, Joseph had a problem: should he treat them as brothers or as strangers? Should he be vindictive or not? The second time, the problem was resolved in his mind. They are my brothers, we are one family, one household, one group—regardless of their behavior of so many years ago. When he was drunk, in complete confusion, he forgot the charges that they were spies—there was no more problem. A stream of great, passionate love replaced Joseph's anger against them and his

[handwritten margin note at top: → No longer be haunted, dominated by? ~ And God "remembered"]

memories of years ago, when they had practiced chicanery against him. Joseph, though he knew the whole time who the brothers were, found love in his heart for them. "They drank and became intoxicated with him" (Gen. 43:34): it was not logical, but there was a change of personality and of memory. Joseph forgot the sale. The change moved Joseph from acting as the tyrant of the land into a state of brotherliness. Earlier, the brothers had told Jacob, What can we do? Do you expect sympathy on the part of the tyrant? You could not expect that from this stranger. The second time the brothers came, Joseph knew very well that he would not punish them, and he decided in favor of not simply mercy and pardon, but of reconciliation with them as brothers.

Of course, the brothers should have understood. Why else would an Egyptian viceroy give a reception for the brothers of Joseph, announce their names in accordance with their age, present them with gifts, and bless Benjamin? After all, Zebulun was a merchant—he was not a fool; Issachar was a scholar; he too was not a fool. Simeon and Levi were not fools. Where was their common sense? Apparently, they "were intoxicated with him." Their intellects did not operate. They did not know that he was Joseph. Was it so difficult to put two and two together? They could have found out his identity if they had thought reasonably, but they did not.

Joseph—the clever, intelligent, and cautious ruler who had saved the Egyptian empire from starvation—acted like a drunk. He was so overcome that he decided to not be vindictive; because of the Almighty's intervention it became possible for him to forget all the experiences he had lived through. Joseph was not bothered by the past anymore, because "they drank" and lost their minds. In Biblical Hebrew there is an expression "shekhurat ve-lo mi-yayin, drunken, but not with wine" (Is. 51:21); shikkor can mean lacking the power of thinking, of arriving at conclusions, of identifying people. It was a night of rec-

[handwritten margin note at bottom: → what does "forget" mean here?]

onciliation between brother and brother which was about to end at the crack of dawn.

"As morning dawned" (Gen. 44:3), the fantastic experience of Joseph with regard to the brothers was forgotten. The night was a night of drunken confusion. But with the rising of dawn, Joseph regained his consciousness and his memory moved toward the earlier experience, giving rise to the urge of vindictiveness.

The verse states, "As morning dawned, *ha-anashim shullehu,* the men were sent away." Not "morning dawned and *Joseph's brothers* were sent away"—they were *anashim* again. If the Torah had said *"nishlehu,"* it would have meant that Joseph sent them away with an assignment. *Shullehu* means they were simply removed, expelled. When the dawn began to rise, they were not brothers anymore; they were strange *anashim* who had no right to be in the viceroy's palace. The *anashim* were thrown out by Joseph's security guard, and he forbade them to enter the grounds—an act of complete alienation between Joseph and the brothers. There were no kisses and presentation of gifts and prayers. There was no outpouring of love toward Benjamin. Once again Joseph was the Egyptian, the cruel face of the tyrant, "the master of the land."

What a difference between the scene at night and the scene at dawn! At night there was love, understanding, and brotherliness; in the morning, accusations, anger, and another excuse to bring them back, because they had stolen the goblet. "The morning dawned and the *anashim* were sent away."

Joseph and Judah

After Joseph's goblet was found in Benjamin's bag, Judah approached Joseph and engaged him in a lengthy debate. The Midrash (Gen. Rabbah 93:2) asked why the other brothers were not concerned with the problem of Benjamin. Why did they not participate in the controversy in support of Judah? The answer was that the other brothers said to themselves: Two kings are engaged in a controversy, and we will not benefit by the victory of either party. Intuitively, they felt that the controversy did not revolve about their young brother Benjamin, but about Jewish historical destiny, that is, about whose descendant would be the King Messiah—Joseph's or Judah's.

Joseph wanted to be king, to combine political and economic power with spiritual leadership. He dreamt of sheaves and he also dreamt of stars. Judah was not a dreamer. Yet apparently there was something in his personality which commanded respect and obedience. Judah was always in front. When Joseph was sold, it was at the suggestion of Judah. And now Judah is in the forefront; he is the one who argues with Joseph. It was he who had the courage to argue with an Egyptian tyrant at whose mercy they stood. He was a very strong and powerful personality who radiated authority. "*Gur aryeh Yehudah*, Judah is a lion cub" (Gen. 49:9).

Joseph lost the battle because he showed weakness. If Joseph had controlled himself, the brothers would have been compelled to return to Canaan without Benjamin. Jacob would never have left Benjamin in Egypt alone; he would have come to plead on behalf of Benjamin; doing so, he would have prostrated himself before Joseph not once but seven times, the way he did before Esau. Joseph's dream of everyone bowing to him would have been fulfilled. But "Joseph could not restrain himself before all his attendants, and he cried, 'Cause all men to go out before me,' and he wept aloud. . . . And Joseph said unto his brothers, 'I am Joseph' " (Gen. 45:1, 3).

The very moment that Joseph disclosed his identity, he ceased to be a ruler as far as his brothers were concerned. From then on, Joseph was not viceroy of Egypt but the talented lad of Jacob's house. Who was going to prostrate himself before this Joseph? He lost the kingdom. He was too gentle, too good, too fine. Jewish history took a different turn.

Why did Providence will that Joseph should lose and Judah win? We study the Bible as the book of destiny, determining not only a story of events that transpired thirty-five hundred years ago, but a story of events that are transpiring now and which will transpire in the future. Why, then, did Joseph lose the final battle?

In order to grasp the rationale for this strange drama, we must retrace the story of Jacob. Laban had two daughters, Leah and Rachel. The Bible attests to Rachel's beauty; she was "beautiful in form and pleasant to behold" (Gen. 29:17). Leah was not attractive. Jacob loved Rachel very much and he told Laban that he was ready to serve seven years for her. Rachel certainly knew of Jacob's love for her and reciprocated.

How, then, could she acquiesce to the scheme devised by Laban to substitute Leah for her? How could she forgo her love for and devotion to Jacob? A young girl who is in love with a young boy—is there an emotion which is more powerful or more committing than such a love? How could she tolerate defeat in such a matter? Our talmudic scholars tell us (*Megillah* 13b) that not only did she not tell Jacob about the plans of her father, but she cooperated with him and her sister in the conspiracy, betraying the secret password she had with Jacob. Why did Rachel participate in this deceit?

I believe the answer is plain. The covenantal community that God established with Abraham displayed two characteristic moral streaks, two tendencies which *prima facie* are contradictory and mutually exclusive. First, the covenantal community does not shrink from power. We have never endorsed the Christian claim that the meek will inherit the earth. Throughout the Bible people fought for power, strength, and independence. Without power, one cannot be majestic and dignified. Majesty and dignity are not sinful, they are moral virtues.

Of course, the majesty and dignity of the human being expresses itself in the fact that man has inalienable rights, including the basic right to engage in productive and gainful work, to be able to hold onto the fruit of his work. Human beings have a moral right to defend their possessions and, if necessary, to fight for them. Man is not a slave.

Judaism has always thought highly of work. God Himself works, as the first chapter of Genesis tells us. God did not redeem us from work; He redeemed us from slavery, from not being able to appreciate the fruits of our labor. The patriarchs were working, productive people. Abraham was very rich in cattle and possessed silver and gold. He was able to protect his rights and defend himself against any onslaught. He declared war on the five kings in order to free Lot. The dignity of man expresses itself through his ability to take a stand and to defend whatever God has given him, to defy opponents if their opposition is wrong. Self-affirmation is a relevant trait of man in general and of the covenantal community in particular.

However, the covenantal community displays another trait as well: sacrificial action, the ability to give away and to renounce basic inalienable rights for the sake of a great vision, an ideal, or for the benefit of another human being or community. Abraham, who was dedicated to his daily pursuits as a shepherd and a trader, who accumulated wealth, was ready to give everything away. The story of the *Akedah* tells us about the readiness of our patriarch to sacrifice everything, including his only child. Covenantal man knows when to act like a warrior—majestic, dignified, and proud—and when to part with everything he has.

This dialectic, this thesis and antithesis, revolves about two *middot* of the Holy One: *hesed* and *gevurah*, kindness and strength, or expansion and contraction. Sometimes the Almighty reveals Himself through the medium of *gevurah* and at other times through the medium of *hesed*, so human beings walk in the footsteps of their Creator. Man must know the secret of when to retreat into his private four cubits and shut the gates, so to say, and when he should tear down the fences and the barriers and live an open life. It is paradoxical, but this is Judaism.

Leah and Rachel were not merely people. Leah was the personification of *middat ha-gevurah*, of dignity and majesty. God wanted her to fight for her elementary rights. Usually, the meanings of biblical names are very important. The name Leah is derived from the root *lamed-alef-hei*, to be tired, to work hard. For example, "*Ve-nil'u*, Egypt grew weary of trying to drink water from the River" (Ex. 7:18). They tried to somehow get some water and finally they failed. "And now when it befalls you, *va-teleh*, you become weary" (Job 4:5). The very first time you face a test and conquer a challenge, you are already exhausted.

A person who has no responsibilities can never enjoy the great experience of being fatigued and tired after a good day's constructive work. Leah is a woman who is burdened with many responsibilities and conscientiously discharges them. Leah represents self-assertion and constructive work to the point of exhaustion and fatigue. The mere fact that she consented to Laban's scheme demonstrates that she was courageous, for she had what to fear. Jacob could have thrown her out on her ear. That she agreed to such an adventurous undertaking shows courage and valor. She was courageous in her handling of matters and was capable of defending her rights. Isn't a young woman, even if she is not attractive, entitled to marry a young man? God granted Leah weak eyes in order to make her display her resoluteness and articulateness. She symbolized the strength of Jewish character and the unshakable will of the Jew throughout the ages and millennia. It is because of that persistence, that stubbornness and tenacity, that we still remain a living people after thirty-five hundred years of persecution and massacres.

Rachel is the opposite of Leah. She is the tragic heroine who lives for others and not for herself. She gave up her most precious possessions and her elementary rights in order to make it possible for others to find the happiness denied them. Rachel represents *hesed*. A young girl who was in love with a boy gives up her fondest dreams for the sake of an older, unattractive sister. She helped her sister take Jacob away from herself. She brushed aside all her own hopes and cherished wishes because her sister was also entitled to the same happiness which Providence had showered upon her, but denied to her sister.

Rachel means a lamb. In the Bible, the lamb is the symbol of a mute animal that does not complain: "He was persecuted and afflicted, but he did not open his mouth; like a lamb being led to the slaughter or a ewe that is silent before her shearers, he did not open his mouth" (Is. 53:7). True, we do hear her complain once: "Give me children, or else I die" (Gen. 30:1). We have never heard her complain until now; all of a sudden, in distress and despair at being barren and condemned to loneliness for the rest of her life, she exploded. After all, she was a human being; there was a limit to her ability to tolerate distress and suffering. It was not a complaint; it was the shriek of helplessness.

Leah represented *gevurah*, and Judah was a son of Leah. Judah's personality radiated power, authority, and prestige. As Jacob described him, Judah crouched as a lion, and "who shall dare rouse him?" (Gen. 49:9) The Kotzker Rebbe read it: Judah is a lion not only when he stands upright, but even when he falls, even though he makes a mistake. Who would rouse Judah from his fall? No one could have helped him rise again but he himself. Judah is self-asserting, valiant, and fearless; he personifies dignity and majesty.

In the sixth chapter of his *Shemonah Perakim*, Maimonides describes two moral types. One is the *kovesh et yitzro,* one who controls his instinctual urges but is not immune to temptation. No matter how lion-like Judah was, he yielded to temptation. On two occasions, he failed miserably to meet the challenge of the horror that confronted him; he acted not like a fearless lion but like a coward. Yet he rose all by himself, without anyone else extending a helping hand. He sinned, but he repented beautifully and heroically with an open mind and contrite heart. In the incident with Tamar, he was not embarrassed to confess publicly, to admit the truth in front of all his friends and associates by saying the unforgettable words, *"Tzadekah mimmenni, She is more righteous than I"* (Gen. 38:26). He was not a natural saint, but the moment he failed, he had the superhuman valor to rise again. The *Mekhilta* in *Beshalah* (*Vayehi* 5) tells us that the disciples of R. Tarfon asked their master: Why did Judah win the battle against Joseph and become the king? It was because he had a lion's heart. Therefore, his descendant Nahshon the son of Amminadab and the rest of the tribe of Judah were the first to jump into the Red Sea when it split. How much firmness and majestic fearlessness did Judah exhibit when he argued with Joseph about Benjamin! After all, the Egyptian viceroy could do anything to him. But the lion's heart was roused and he was ready to fight. In a word, his shibboleth was *gevurah*.

Joseph belonged to a different moral group, the *hasidim* who are moral by inclination, people over whom sin has no power. The Satan has no access to them; their lives are not stormy. They do not display the heroism of rising again, because they never fall. They walk along a straight path; they do not roll down a steep incline into an abyss, nor do they perform the miracle of stopping the downward movement at the brink of the cleft. Joseph never sinned; he resisted the charm of the vulgar Egyptian woman.

Jacob and Moses bestowed the title of saintliness upon Joseph, *"nezir ehav"* (Gen. 49:26, Deut. 33:16). Joseph was the son of Rachel, to whom was assigned a mission to sacrifice, to retreat from positions won with blood and tears. He was the talented boy, and because of his talents he was sold into slavery. He retreated many times, thus sacrificing himself, but his real sacrifice was the way he treated his brothers when they were at his mercy: "Be not grieved, nor angry with yourselves, that you sold me here" (Gen. 45:5). He was not the least bit vindictive.

Only a son of Rachel could have done that. Only the son of Rachel, who had sacrificed her love for Leah's sake, could downgrade his own self and offer friendship and kindness to his brothers who were responsible for all the misery and agony he had experienced. Joseph was the representative of *hesed* and *kedushah*.

Who then should be the king: the representative of *gevurah* or the representative of *hesed* and *kedushah*? The problem was submitted to the Almighty, and He decided in favor of *gevurah*. The king is the trustee and leader of the people; he must possess all facets of *gevurah*: the ability to acquire, to defend, to possess, and to protect. Sacrificial life is good as far as the individual is concerned. But the king cannot be a sacrificial type at the expense of the nation.

David could be a king. He resembled Judah; he, too, ascended to the greatest heights and then fell into an abyss. Yet he managed, like Judah, to rise again to still greater heights. David is the great teacher of *teshuvah*, repentance. Only the ruler who encounters sin, who falls for short intervals but who also knows the art of rising, of lifting himself up—only he will understand his people and have compassion for the unfortunate ones who strayed, for those who got lost and fell. The saint would have no understanding of sin and error; the sacrificial soul is too sensitive to insist, to demand, and to defend.

Joseph lost the kingship because he could not control himself; his emotions were overflowing, and he had too much love in his bosom. When Jacob came to Egypt, he beheld not some pagan Egyptian tyrant, but his beloved son Joseph, before whom he would never prostrate himself in acknowledgment of kingship. Providence had finally rendered the decision in the controversy between Judah and Joseph: Judah was declared the winner. He understood that people were frail and that from time to time they would sin. He knew that sinners should not be barred from reaching out for *teshuvah*; they should be helped to get up and rise again to greater heights.

Joseph did not win the kingship; Judah did. That is exactly how "the light of the Messiah" emerges from the sale of Joseph. When Joseph was sold, the problem was the identity of the Messiah—is he to be a descendant of Joseph or a descendant of Judah? That is what the Midrash means when it says that when Joseph was sold into slavery, "The Almighty was busy preparing the light of the Messiah" (Gen. Rabbah 85:1). The process of selecting the Messiah commenced on the day of the sale of Joseph. The winner of the conflict was Judah and not Joseph.

Wagons to Jacob

When the brothers returned to their father, "They spoke to him all the words of Joseph which he had said unto them; and when he saw the wagons (*agalot*) which Joseph had sent to bear him, the spirit of Jacob their father revived" (Gen. 45:27).

Of course, the question is, why did Jacob accept their story after he had seen the wagons? They had repeated words that Joseph had told them to pass on to their father. Yet Jacob was skeptical; he did not believe it was true. If so, why did he change his mind after he noticed the wagons which allegedly were sent by Joseph?

Rashi (s.v. *et*) asked this question and made the following observation: As evidence that it was he who had sent the message, Joseph instructed them to tell Jacob that at the time he left Jacob, they were studying the laws of *eglah arufah*, the laws pertaining to the heifer whose neck is broken. It is to this that Scripture refers when saying, "And he saw the *agalot* that Joseph sent." The wagons were sent by Pharaoh, not Joseph; Jacob saw something else—Joseph's reference to the heifer.

The section of *eglah arufah* deals with the Jewish concept of the responsibility of the leaders of a community. If someone is found slain and it is not known who murdered him, the nearest city is duty bound to bring down a heifer to a rough valley (or a brook). There they are supposed to break the neck of the heifer and say: "Our hands have not shed this blood, nor have our eyes seen it; forgive, O Lord!" (Deut. 21:7–8) We all know the question which was raised by the Mishnah (*Sotah* 9:6): "Could it have come into our mind that the elders of the court were shedders of blood? What the Bible means is: We did not send him away without food, nor did we see him journeying and leaving with none to accompany him."

It is almost frightening how demanding the Torah is concerning the leadership that goes hand in hand with power. It is a responsibility that encompasses not only direct action but indirect—in fact, very removed—action. Of course, the leader is responsible for all his actions. His judgment must be right; he must not accept bribes; he must act in accordance with the principles of justice and charity. However, he is also charged with responsibility for things and events that are, *prima facie*, very far removed from his concerns and interests. The people wielding power are the ones responsible for and guilty of the crime.

Jacob knew that Joseph was destined to be a mighty man, that power would be concentrated in his hands (Gen. 37:11). He continued studying with Joseph the morality of leadership and power.

When Jacob heard Joseph's message, he wondered: Is the old Joseph still alive? The fact that Joseph was Jacob's son biologically did not satisfy Jacob. Jacob was searching not only for his son but for his disciple. He assumed that a man who served as ruler of Egypt had been assimilated into the general pagan society. He did not believe that Joseph could have preserved his spiritual identity and remained loyal to all the teachings he had received during his seventeen years with Jacob. Of course, when they told him about the last lesson Jacob and Joseph had shared together, he realized that Joseph had survived years of torture in exile; he had remained his son and disciple. Jacob said: I do not need any more evidence. My son Joseph is indeed alive.

Not only was his son alive; when he saw the wagons, he realized that the brothers' story—that Joseph was second to the king—was true as well. I believe that the wagons convinced Jacob for a simple reason. Egypt in antiquity was a highly developed industrial power, an exceptionally advanced country in matters of technology and manufacture. Egypt tamed and domesticated the horse and turned it into a war-animal, as Hannibal did with the elephant. Their chariots were famous throughout the Mideast; together with the horse, they constituted an almost invincible might. "And the Egyptians pursued and came after them to the midst of the sea; even all Pharaoh's chariots and his horsemen" (Ex. 14:23).

Apparently, wagons were manufactured in Egypt exclusively under the auspices and imprimatur of the king. Most probably, the purpose of manufacturing wagons was a military one. The *agalot* accompanied the chariots for the transportation of freight, ammunition, food, and so forth, and were quite probably under the strict control of Pharaoh. No one could sell or send them abroad without Pharaoh's specific permission.

I believe that the Torah pointed this out. When Pharaoh heard the news that Joseph's brothers had come, he told Joseph, "Say to your brothers: Load your animals . . . and take your father and your households and come to me" (Gen. 45:17–18). There was no command, just a suggestion. However, in the following verse Pharaoh changes his request into a command: "Now you are commanded, this do, take you wagons out of the land of Egypt for your little ones, for your wives, and bring your father, and come." Why the sudden change from suggestion to command? It was because the wagons could be taken out of Egypt only if the king issued a formal order to do so. Pharaoh said: I hereby instruct you to take the wagons out of the land of Egypt. When Joseph sent the wagons, he did it upon the specific orders issued by Pharaoh. A formal command to that effect had to be released. When Jacob saw the wagons that Joseph sent, he realized immediately that Joseph was close to the king. An ordinary person could not have done that.

However, there is more to the wagons than meets the eye. We read, "And the rumor thereof was heard in Pharaoh's house, saying, Joseph's brothers have come; and it was good in the eyes of Pharaoh and in the eyes of his servants" (Gen. 45:16). Why did Pharaoh and his servants welcome the news about the arrival of Joseph's brothers? What difference did it make to them whether or not Joseph found his brothers?

Nahmanides (s.v. *ve-ta'am*) gave the following answer: The social elite of Egypt could not tolerate the fact that a former prisoner was second to Pharaoh. The Egyptian aristocracy felt hurt by the fact that an ex-convict, a dark and mysterious figure who had escaped from his native land, ruled Egypt. Now, they discovered that Joseph was a scion of a great, noble family. Apparently, the renown of Abraham as the Prince of God had spread over the whole Mideast. Pharaoh is happy that his vizier is a grandson of that mysterious Abraham.

I believe that there was something else that caused Pharaoh to show interest in the brothers of Joseph. Pharaoh admired Joseph. He understood and fully appreciated Joseph's genius as organizer, executive, and planner, on the one hand, and as visionary blessed with a creative imagination, on the other. In fact, as stated earlier, Joseph's greatness consisted in the dialectic, in the duality within his personality. Joseph was a dreamer, a visionary blessed with fantasy and power of anticipation. On the other hand, he was a tough, down-to-earth, pragmatic utilitarian, a realist and a fact-conscious executive. He was a dreamer and a dream-interpreter at the same time. This combination of *phantasia* and *pragmos* is very rare. Fortunate is the country blessed with such a person. Joseph saved the entire Mideast from the disaster of famine. Pharaoh, as an enlightened ruler, saw all this and was immensely thankful to Joseph.

However, one person, no matter how great and dynamic, does not suffice. Many great men are necessary. Pharaoh thought that a family into which a great man of Joseph's caliber was born must have more talented people, more creative minds.

Perhaps all twelve were blessed with charisma, imagination, and practical sense. He could not understand why Joseph had never asked him for permission to bring his family to Egypt. Joseph's antagonists maligned him by circulating the rumor that the grand vizier was not a loyal citizen of Egypt: His loyalties are divided, his allegiance qualified. He does not look upon Egypt as his ultimate home. He treats Egypt as a stopover station of temporary significance only. His home is in Canaan. That is why he has not attempted to urge his family to settle in Egypt.

Pharaoh did not believe these accusations. However, he waited impatiently for the reunion of Joseph and his clan and the final decision to settle in Egypt. Suddenly Pharaoh heard the good news. The reconciliation has taken place. They are here. Many times he had discussed it with Joseph. The latter told him that he could not inform his father and the members of his family that he was alive and successful. Joseph told him about a covenant which he did not understand, about the ability of the Hebrews to wait patiently for the event to take place. Joseph waited for God's intervention; he refused to accelerate the historical unfolding of destiny.

Pharaoh could not grasp Joseph's philosophy, but he had great confidence in him. Now, he thought, this strange and talented family will be integrated into Egyptian society, which will avail itself of the rare capabilities of these immigrants from Canaan. The invitation he issued was most generous. Pharaoh was in an ecstatic mood. The invitation represents not only generosity but enthusiasm, as if this event were the most relevant one in the history of his kingdom. Indeed, the presence of the Jew in a country has always been a blessing to society. No country was ever impoverished or lost its economic prominence because of the Jew.

However, Pharaoh said something very enigmatic. Pharaoh emphasized time and again that they must bring Jacob to Egypt. By implication, he conveyed to the brothers an ultimatum that they must not come to Egypt without Jacob (Gen. 45:17–19). From the affirmative, one concludes the negative. The invitation was extended mainly to Jacob. I do not want your presence without him. Jacob must join you.

Pharaoh had a great understanding of spirituality. We know that Joseph's presence had an enormous impact upon him. Joseph humanized and sensitized him. He succeeded in making Egypt the provider of food for the Mideast without discriminating between Egyptians and foreigners. There was a humanitarian aspect to the distribution system introduced by Joseph. The peasants retained eighty percent of the harvest for themselves; only twenty percent was given to the treasury (Gen. 47:24)—a pretty decent agreement for antiquity! Joseph convinced Pharaoh that justice and charity must prevail, that a civilized country cannot exist on technology alone. A moral system is indispensable. In their long conversations, Joseph certainly told Pharaoh about the covenant, about his father, grandfather, and great-grandfather, about the strange community they had established in Canaan, about their way of life, about *hesed* and *mishpat*, about hospitality and visiting the sick, about the *Akedah* and total commitment to the Almighty, who is concerned with man and his way of life. He most probably told him about *imago Dei*.

Pharaoh was intrigued and fascinated by Jacob, and he was eager to meet him. Pharaoh felt that Joseph's talented and brilliant personality had been nurtured by the unique tradition in which he was raised and which had been ingrained in him since infancy. He knew that not only Joseph's spirituality, but also his executive and administrative capacity, would be affected if Joseph decided to sever the ties binding him to his father and the latter's tradition. A beautiful, blossoming tree can thrive only if planted in the proper climate; cold and ice will kill it immediately. The suitable climate for Joseph could be created only by Jacob, who was the source of the beauty that Joseph possessed. The origin of his beauty was the old tradition represented by the old father.

Of course, Pharaoh wanted to have the brothers join Egyptian society and contribute to its growth and development. They most probably resemble Joseph, Pharaoh thought. They are brilliant and competent. However, their roots must drink the waters of Canaan, not those of Egypt. Only if the old man will join them will they succeed here. That was Pharaoh's opinion.

He orders them to bring their father. Of course the father will never assimilate into Egyptian society. You cannot expect a man of his age to feel fully integrated into Egyptian society. Yet the tree will grow and bear fruit. Without Jacob, nothing worthwhile will transpire. That is why Pharaoh wanted Jacob to settle in Egypt.

Reading the story, we come to the conclusion that even though Pharaoh sent the wagons for the children, womenfolk, and Jacob, the main reason for sending them was to please Jacob, to make the traveling easier for Jacob. "Now you are commanded, this you shall do: Take wagons out of the land of Egypt for your little ones and for your wives; and *carry your father* and come" (Gen. 45:19). "When he saw the wagons which Joseph had sent *to carry him*, the spirit of Jacob their father revived" (45:27). "The sons of Israel carried their father Jacob, and their children and their wives in the wagons that Pharaoh had sent *to carry him*" (46:5).

The special emphasis on carrying Jacob—"*u-nesatem et avikhem*," "*laset oto*"—reminds us of the carrying of the Ark and the Tabernacle during the sojourn of the Israelites in the desert. At the dedication of the Tabernacle, the princes donated covered wagons and animals to pull them: "And they brought their offering . . . six covered wagons and twelve oxen, a wagon for two of the princes and for each one an ox" (Num. 7:3). Moses gave the covered wagons and the oxen to Gerson and Merari for their service, namely, for the transportation of the Tabernacle. However, "he did not give [wagons and oxen] to the sons of Kehat, because the service of the holiness was incumbent upon them and they were to bear it upon their shoulders" (ibid. 7:9).

I have the impression that the children and women were transported in the wagons the way the children of Merari and Gerson moved the Tabernacle, the boards, and so on, while Jacob's wagon was pulled or carried by his children. For to move Jacob was a holy service, not inferior to the bearing of the covenantal Ark. No matter how sacred the tablets were, they were nevertheless stone. Jacob was a living sacred being. God's word was part of Jacob's personality. It was engraved not on dead matter but on living tissue, a sensitive soul and a great creative mind. If the stone tablets must not be carried by oxen, then the living tablet certainly must not be pushed by some mechanical force. Moses did not assign wagons to the sons of Kehat because they were performing the holy service and were commanded, therefore, to bear the Ark on their shoulders. The same applies to Jacob. The sons were told to bear him on their shoulders or to push or pull the wagons by hand. For Jacob, like the tablets, personified the exalted, sublime, and divine.

How could an Egyptian tyrant be impressed by the great figure of Jacob, whom he had never met and who preached morals diametrically opposed to those of Egypt? It was Joseph, with his charm and spiritual grandeur, who changed the tyrant into a sensitive person who admired Joseph and his tradition. Pharaoh sent the wagons; however, it was with instructions that represented Joseph's outlook and philosophy. Pharaoh's wagons were indeed Joseph's.

❧ *An Old Father*

Jacob and Joseph

Parashat Vayeshev and *Parashat Vayehi* begin with the number seventeen: "At seventeen years of age Joseph tended the flocks with his brothers" (Gen. 37:2); "Jacob lived in the land of Egypt seventeen years" (Gen. 47:28). This is not a coincidence. Jacob's teachings were responsible for Joseph's tenacity and persistence in times of distress as well as in times of success. However, when Joseph attained the pinnacle of power, determining the fate of millions, he was still young and vigorous. Jacob knew that power corrupts. The longer a leader exercises authority, the tougher, more proud, and less sensitive he becomes. There was still danger that Joseph, after Jacob's death, might imitate the Oriental rulers in their way of life. Jacob had to repeat the teachings he had first passed on to Joseph in the course of his seventeen years of childhood and adolescence. He had to fortify the Joseph, the middle-aged viceroy of Egypt wielding absolute power, against all the temptations associated with the exercise of power. It took the old man seventeen years of continuous teaching, the same number of years during which he had fashioned Joseph's young personality and imbued it with the morality and piety of Abraham and Isaac.

Our Sages say that Joseph was the double of Jacob; his facial features bore a striking resemblance to those of Jacob (*Tanhuma, Vayeshev* 2). Their historical experiences were similar. Abraham and Isaac joined the covenant in the Land of Israel. Jacob and Joseph were the first ones given the task of proving that the covenant can be observed in exile, in a strange land, among a different society whose language and way of life one has to learn. Both were lonely, poor, and foreign. Jacob proved the viability of the covenant outside his homeland by serving Laban for twenty years. Joseph proved in Egypt that one can remain steadfast in his faith in bondage and prison as well as in abundance and power.

A Tradition Maintained

"And the days of Israel's death drew near, and he called his son Joseph and said unto him: If now I have found favor in your sight . . . bury me not, I pray, in Egypt" (Gen. 47:29). The question is obvious: why does the name Jacob occur in the first sentence of this passage (i.e., Gen. 47:28 quoted in the preceding section), while the name Israel appears in the second? In fact, the whole story about the patriarch's request that he be buried in Canaan speaks of him as Israel. Why?

Nahmanides (Gen. 35:10, s.v. *shimkha*; 46:2, s.v. *va-yomer*) already said that, in contradistinction to the change from Abram to Abraham, the name Israel did not replace Jacob. Israel was only added to Jacob. From that moment on, the patriarch is known by two names, Jacob and Israel. Nahmanides explained that the two names reflect two destinies, two roles that the covenantal community plays. Jacob and Israel are not only individual but collective names related to the community as such. We say *Kenesset Yisrael* as well as *Beit Yaakov*.

Our patriarch Jacob was not always an independent individual. He was often subject to someone else, be it a powerful person or a society into whose texture the life of the patriarch was interwoven. The existence of the families of the covenantal community quite often was enmeshed with another existence that stood for the very opposite of what the fathers of the covenant represented.

Jacob spent twenty years in Laban's house, where he worked for Laban like a bondsman. The patriarch's economy was part of Laban's economy. When he returned to Canaan, he was afraid of Esau and tried to allay Esau's vindictiveness by presenting him with a generous gift. Finally, he was compelled to come to Egypt, where the entire household had to adjust itself to the mighty technological civilization.

Whenever the life of the patriarch was appended to another existence, whenever it depended upon extraneous factors, he or the covenantal community appears as Jacob, which signifies dependence, holding on, being pulled along. "And after that his brother came out, his hand grasping the heel of Esau, and he called his name Jacob" (Gen. 25:26). Whenever the patriarch's hand is grasping someone's heel, his appropriate name is Jacob. The latter is not free to determine and mold his destiny.

Israel represents the free Jew, the Jew who has thrown off the chains of subservience and bondage, the proud Jew who engages his enemy in a struggle and defeats him, the Jew who emerges victorious from his engagement with the mysterious antagonist during a long, lonely night. The antagonist admitted that the father of the covenant was victorious: "Your name shall be called no more Jacob, but Israel; for you have contended with God and with men, and have prevailed" (Gen. 32:29). A free, powerful Jew is Israel; a Jew dependent upon others is Jacob.

No wonder that the Bible says *Jacob* lived in Egypt seventeen years. The sojourn of the Jews in Egypt could hardly be considered as a time of glory and dignity. It would have been inappropriate to say that *Israel* lived in the land of Egypt for seventeen years. Where was the power? Where was the freedom? Where was the joy and pride that a free people experiences? The physical sojourn per se is certainly a Jacob experience, one of defeat and humility.

On the other hand, the bondsmen, the slaves beaten by Egypt, humiliated and treated with chicanery and cruelty by their masters, exhibited unusual strength, superhuman tenacity and dedication. They lived in Egypt hundreds of years; they were completely involved in the Egyptian economy. They let themselves be gripped by the land; they became an integral part of Egypt's material civilization. And yet they never gave up completely their spiritual identity, their moral strength, and, particularly, their commitment to the Promised Land. Every one of them knew that at some point in time, a mysterious redeemer would appear who would announce the great message that God had remembered them. All of them waited for the great moment when the good tidings of redemption would be brought to the downtrodden and oppressed. They were physically subservient to their masters, but spiritually proud and independent.

Who implanted in them the faith in redemption, the trust in the *masorah*, the tradition that they would finally return to the land of their fathers as a free covenantal community? It was Jacob! The request he addressed to Joseph that he be buried in the Machpelah Cave instead of having an Egyptian burial plot was considered by Jacob to be of the highest importance. Jacob made Joseph take an oath because burial near his ancestors had great symbolic significance. The memory of that burial would have an almost supernatural impact upon the descendants of Jacob who were born and raised in Egypt. The ceremonial made them aware that their real origin lay elsewhere.

The story about Jacob's will was a reminder to the generations born and educated in Egypt that their real identity was rooted far away from Goshen. It kept alive their commitment to the land. The weak Jacob in exile emerges suddenly as a giant. He succeeded in defeating the Egyptian assimilationist forces; he defeated the old historical rule that a minority must finally succumb to the culture and way of life of the majority. That is why the patriarch expressed his wish not as Jacob, not as a frightened Jew, but as Israel, as the proud Jew fighting with the angels and defying the world. The future of the covenantal people was involved insofar as he spoke as the father of a nation and not merely as an individual.

The Closeness of Generations

However, the perpetuation of the covenantal tradition among the Hebrews required more than the dramatic taking of Jacob's body to the Cave of Machpelah. This alone could not secure the future of Jacob's household. Something more significant was necessary, something representing the very essence of the covenantal community: the closeness of the generations. The covenantal community is a teaching community, not a political community. A teaching community consists not of a young pupil and a young teacher, the way modern theory of education recommends, but of an old teacher—a very old one—and a very young student. The older the teacher, the larger the discrepancy in age, the greater the impact.

We understand very well that an elder, rich in experience and ripe in years, who met the great men of a previous era, is far more capable of transmitting impressions, memories, and feelings. The young pedagogue—who has just heard about events but never witnessed them—cannot enrich the child's imagination and memory as can the old. In a word, the teaching of the *masorah* consists in the art of establishing lines of communication between old and young. Jacob made this possible by symbolically embracing his grandchildren Ephraim and Manasseh and imparting his blessings—that is, the *masorah*— to them directly. In fact, he communicated with Ephraim and Manasseh before he did so with Reuben and Simeon. Generations commune with each other. Ephraim and Manasseh received the tradition directly from Jacob, notwithstanding the pedagogical fact that Joseph should have charged them with responsibility vis-à-vis the tradition. Jacob extended his hand directly to the grandchildren, leaving out Joseph. The communication between old and young is the most characteristic feature of our *masorah*.

Jacob is the father not only of Joseph, but of Ephraim and Manasseh as well. He embraced his grandchildren. Joseph understood the secret of the *masorah* and tried to emulate Jacob. "And Joseph saw the children of the third generation of Ephraim; also the children of Machir the son of Manasseh were born on Joseph's knees" (Gen. 50:23). In other words, Joseph built a bridge spanning the abyss of generations. He felt as close to the third generation as he was to his own children. In the chronology of *masorah*, the transmission of the Abrahamic blessing was a direct one from Jacob to Ephraim and Manasseh and from Joseph to the children of the third generation. Joseph outdid his father. He reached out one generation further than did Jacob.

A Personal Recollection

By sheer association, I recall an experience of my early youth. I was then about seven or eight years old. I attended *heder* in Khaslavich, a small town on the border of White Russia and Russia proper. My father was the rabbi of the town. My teacher was a "*Habadnik*," a follower of the Lubavitcher Rebbe. He was not a great scholar. However, I have been grateful to him all my life because he taught me something which no one else (perhaps with the exception of my mother) taught me. He did not train my mind but somehow addressed himself to my soul and to my heart. Many people practice Judaism but do so in an unimaginative fashion; they lack sweep and depth. He showed me how to behold a vision and how to make it come to life. Not many *heder* boys knew how to behold a vision and certainly not how to make it real. He taught me how to dream, how to experience Judaism and not just practice it.

The episode that I am about to relate took place on a murky winter day in January. I still remember the day; it was cloudy and overcast. It was after the Hanukkah festival, and the Torah portion of the week was *Vayigash* (Gen. 44:18–47:27). With the end of Hanukkah, the little serenity which this festival brought into the monotonous and listless lives of these poor Jews passed. Most of them were poor peddlers in that small town on the river Sozh (a tributary of the Dnieper). As far as the boys from the *heder* were concerned, a long and desolate winter lay ahead. It was a period in which we had to get up while it was still dark and then return home with lanterns in our hands because nightfall was so early.

On that particular day, all the boys were in a depressed mood—listless, lazy, and sad. We recited—or I would rather say chanted mechanically—the first sentences of *Parashat Vayigash* in a dull monotone. We read mechanically: "Then Judah approached him [Joseph] and said: . . . My lord asked his servants saying: 'Have you a father or a brother?' And we said to my lord: 'We have an old father, an *av zaken*, and a young child of his old age, a *yeled zekunim*' " (44:19–20).

Then something strange happened. The *melammed*, the teacher, who was half asleep while the boy was droning on the words in Yiddish and in Hebrew, suddenly jumped to his feet with a strange, enigmatic gleam in his eyes. He leaped to his feet like a lion. He usually had velvety blue eyes, but suddenly his eyes became piercing, searching, and investigating. He motioned to the reader to stop and turned to me, *"Podrabin!"*— assistant to the rabbi, as he called me whenever he was excited—"What kind of question did Joseph ask his brothers? 'Do you have a father?' Of course they have a father; everybody has a father! The only person who had no father was the first man of creation, Adam. But whoever is born into this world has a father. What kind of question was it?"

I tried to answer. "Joseph," I finally said, "meant to find out whether the father was still alive." "In such a case," the *melammed* thundered back at me, "he should have phrased the question differently: Is your father still alive?" (cf. Gen. 43:27). To argue with the *melammed* was useless. As he began to speak, he no longer addressed himself to the boys. The impression he gave was that he was speaking to some mysterious visitor, a guest who had come into the *heder*, into that cold room.

"Joseph did not intend to ask his brothers about *avot de-itgalin!*" (I later discovered that this was a Habad term for parenthood which is open and visible.) "He was asking them about *avot de-itkasin*, about the mysterious, the hidden and invisible parenthood." In modern idiom, I would say he meant to express the fact that Joseph inquired about existential parenthood and not biological parenthood.

"Joseph," the *melammed* continued with fervor, "was anxious to know whether they felt themselves committed to their roots, to their origins. Are you, Joseph asked the brothers, rooted in your father? Do you look upon him the way the branches or blossoms look upon the roots of the tree? Do you look upon your father as the foundation of your existence? Do you see him as a provider and sustainer of your existence? Or are you a band of rootless shepherds who forget their *makor*, their origin, and wander from place to place, from pasture to pasture?"

Suddenly, he stopped addressing himself to the strange visitor and he began to talk to us. Raising his voice, he asked: "Are you modest and humble? Do you admit that the old father represents an old tradition? Do you believe that the father is capable of telling you something new, something exciting, something challenging, something you did not know before? Or are you insolent, arrogant, and vain, denying your dependence upon your father and your *makor*?"

"Do you have a father?!" exclaimed the *melammed*, pointing at my study-mate Yitzik, who was considered the town's prodigy. The *melammed* turned to him and said: "What do you say? Who knows more, you or your father the blacksmith who can hardly read Hebrew? Are you proud, Yitzik, of your father," he asked. "Do you feel humble in his presence? Do you have a father?"

And then he ended in a whisper, "If a Jew admits to the supremacy of his father, then he admits to the supremacy of the Universal Father, who is very old, *Atik Yomin, me-olam ad olam!*"

This is the experience I had with my *melammed*. I have never forgotten it.

We may interpret Joseph's second question in a similar manner. When Joseph asked, "Do you have a brother?" he was not really interested in whether they had a biological brother who had inherited the identical genetic code from their parents. Joseph wanted to know: Does your time awareness and your existential awareness embrace only you and your friends, your parents and children, or does this "I exist" awareness embrace generations yet unborn as well? Do you believe that the future can be shaped by our present actions? Do you know that it is worthwhile to work and sacrifice for the future that is represented by this little brother? Or do you know nothing of the future—nothing of the little boy and nothing of the old man?

Both questions asked by Joseph were answered in the affirmative: Yes, we do have a very old father in whom we feel that we all are deeply rooted—and we are rooted in the eternal ideals of all fathers, in the *Atik Yomin*. And yes, we also have a wonderful, young, talented, bright child with shining eyes, who represents the world of tomorrow. We have the feeling, when we glance at the child, that he is challenging us to make possible the birth of generations yet unborn, to help nonbeing emerge as something real.

The answer the sons of Jacob gave to Joseph must hold true even today. We are still committed to our "old father," to a great mysterious past and to eternal ideals. Only this can account for our mourning for a Temple consumed by fire nearly two thousand years ago; only this can account for our deep attachment to the Land of Israel. We are committed not only to a great past, but to a glorious future, to the "young child." The child is our ambassador of the future. We behold a great vision of tomorrow, and we know that in order to realize it we must know how to bring up and educate the child. We are both past-minded and future-oriented.

Judaism demands that we arrange a rendezvous between the old father and the young child; this is the *masorah*, the tradition, the oral transmission, the merging of past and future. The *av zaken* must teach the *yeled zekunim* two things: divine discipline and divine romance.

Moses, in his farewell address to the people, said, "You shall know in your heart that just as a father disciplines his son, so the Lord your God disciplines you; and you shall observe the commandments of the Lord your God, to walk in His ways and to fear Him" (Deut. 8:5–6). The Torah teaches the Jew to live a disciplined life, a life following specific rules, a life with sequence and continuity, a life provided with orderliness. The main distinction between Judaism and paganism consists in the fact that paganism preaches an orgiastic, hypnotic life, while Judaism demands sacrificial action and the capacity for resignation. As we know from the story of the Tree of Knowledge, the test of a human being is whether he can discipline himself, whether he yields to temptation or overcomes it.

There is a second disciplined action which the *av zaken* must teach the young child: discipline with regard to human relations. While disciplined carnal action leads to sanctity, disciplined social action leads to honesty, to *emet* and *hesed*. Disciplined social action commands the respect of the non-Jew and leads to dignity. The question of whether I am entitled to the profit which is offered me is just as important as the inquiry into whether the chicken is *treif* or kosher. The traditional community will exist or disappear by our observance of these *mitzvot*. We will exist if we command dignity by practicing charity, honesty, and truthfulness. And we will lose the battle if we employ methods which are beneath the dignity of any Jew.

There is also a third kind of discipline which the *av zaken* must teach the young child, namely, a disciplined inner life. The

Torah is not interested only in human physical actions—be it on an individual physiological level such as eating, be it on the social level such as manufacturing or selling goods. The Torah is also interested in the inner activities of the Jew, in his emotional life. The Torah knows very well that some emotions that a person experiences, such as hate and envy, are disjunctive, and the Torah requires the person to disown such emotions, to reject them and drive them out of his personality. If an emotion is destructive, then man is capable of rejecting it.

Let me give you a personal example. I was very envious as a child. I was envious of my friends, because they did not consider me a bright child. This impression was created because I was intellectually honest. I would declare that I did not comprehend a topic when I did not truly understand it. I was very envious of another child in *heder*, who was reputed to know one hundred pages of the Talmud by heart. I remember my father called me in once and told me that envy is a *middah megunah*, a deplorable trait, a bad habit, an emotional enemy. These emotions have been forbidden by the Torah: "*Lo tahmod*, You shall not covet" (Ex. 20:14) and "*Lo tit'aveh*, You shall not desire" (Deut. 5:18). I began to train myself to overcome my envy, and I succeeded. Now there is no envy in my heart. On the contrary, I rejoice in the success of my fellow man. The Torah demanded of man to integrate into his personality constructive, cathartic emotions such as sympathy, love, and gratitude. One has freedom not only to control his physical acts but also to control his emotional life.

There is yet a fourth discipline which is also important: disciplined thought, how to conceptualize and define, how to understand, abstract, and classify.

However, besides the disciplines which the *av zaken* teaches the *yeled zekunim*, he must teach the child something else: the romance of Judaism, how to experience and to feel it. True, we start with discipline on all levels: carnal, social, emotional, and intellectual. But above all we must teach our children how to live Judaism. Judaism is a norm to be implemented by action, a concept to be analyzed and understood by the intellect, and also a romance to be experienced, lived, and enjoyed. I believe it is the greatest pleasure to study the Torah and to delve into its depths. A new world appears, new horizons. The most exciting of all adventures is to study and think like a Jew. It is the most cleansing, purging, and cathartic of all occupations. The *av zaken* teaches the *yeled zekunim* how to live and experience Judaism.

If we teach well, we will all be able to answer Joseph's question. Yes, we have an old father; yes, we have a young brother.

"You Shall Carry Up My Bones from Here"
Before his death, Joseph gathered his brothers and asked to be buried in the land of Canaan:

> Joseph said to his brothers, "I shall die; and God will surely remember you (*pakod yifkod*), and bring you out of this land unto the land which He swore to Abraham, to Isaac, and to Jacob." And Joseph made the children of Israel take an oath, saying, "God will surely remember you (*pakod yifkod*), and you shall carry up my bones from here" (Gen. 50:24–25).

Why is Joseph's request to be buried in Israel formulated in two verses? The first verse is a statement, an assertion or judgment: "God will surely remember you, and bring you out of this land." Then, in the second verse, "Joseph made the children of Israel"—not his brothers—"take an oath."

I believe that the interpretation is very simple. First, Joseph made a statement to his brothers just before his death. Four generations had already been born in Egypt. Brothers, he said, you know how worried we were about the future of the Jewish community in Egypt after many successful years of sojourning. You know how concerned we were about the destiny of the people. We did not know whether we would win or lose the battle against assimilation; perhaps we would disappear in the melting pot of Egypt. We did not know what the future held in store for us. Now I can tell you, we won the battle. The fourth generation is growing up in dedication and consecration to the Almighty. We will never forget the covenant. For if the fourth generation can do so, the tenth can as well. Their covenantal memory and their moral sensitivity are reassuring, and no matter how far we are from that exalted moment of redemption, no matter how far we are from that great moment when the redeemer will finally appear, I am sure and I can trust that the covenantal community will survive. And when the great redeemer comes, he will find a community ready for him.

When he said "I shall die," he was telling them, I can die with peace of mind, reassured by history that the miracle of the preservation of our identity under the most difficult circumstances has already taken place. We all contributed to this. I too have a share in it, and therefore I have the right not only to ask a favor of my brothers, but to demand, not only from my brothers, but from the entire nation, from the entire community. I have a right to force you to take an oath that my bones will be taken to the Promised Land. That is why the Torah said, "Joseph made the *children of Israel* take an oath."

Just as Jacob's burial in the Promised Land symbolizes that the Jew is just a sojourner in Egypt and belongs somewhere else, so the burial of Joseph's remains in Canaan will have the same symbolic significance—perhaps a greater significance. He did not ask a favor from his brothers, but he demanded it from the people as a community, as a nation. He wanted to be buried in Canaan like Jacob before him. He wanted to demonstrate the truth that no matter how high an office a Jew might hold in Egypt, no matter how famous and powerful and prominent the Jew is in the general society, his spiritual identity does not change. He belongs to the covenantal community. Of course, his steadfastness as a son of the covenant does not conflict with his political loyalty to the state he serves. But on the other hand, the state itself cannot demand from him that he give up his Jewish identity. We believe that we can commit ourselves at a political level to the state or the society in which we live and to the people among whom we live. We can commit ourselves to discharge our duty in the most perfect manner while not sacrificing our Jewish identity. Joseph had shown that. But at the same time that he was very loyal and steadfast as a citizen, his devotion as a citizen did not conflict with his determination to retain his Jewish identity.

Joseph and Moses

Joseph's oath was directed to the entire nation as a demand; he did not appoint any specific executor. Who, then, executed this testament? "Moses took the bones of Joseph with him" (Ex. 13:19). It was the grandchild of Levi.

According to tradition, Levi and Simeon were the two who "conspired against him [i.e., Joseph] to slay him" (Gen. 37:18). Levi was convinced that Joseph was a menace to the house of Jacob; he was so critical of Joseph that he thought the only way to save *Kenesset Yisrael* was to kill him.

Why, then, should his great-grandchild revere Joseph to such an extent? Why would Moses hold up the Exodus on the night of Passover? Suddenly Moses disappeared. Everybody was ready to march, but Moses was not to be found. The Midrash tells us: " 'By night on my bed'—this is the night of Egypt; 'I sought him whom my soul loves'—this is Moses; 'I sought him, but I found him not' " (Song Rabbah 3:1). According to the Midrash, they sent out scouts to find Moses: "I will rise now, and go around in the city; in the markets and in the broad streets will I seek him whom my soul loves; I sought him, but I found him not" (Song 3:2). What was Moses doing at that time? He was searching for Joseph's coffin. He held up the Exodus of six hundred thousand Jews, with the Divine Presence ready to march in front of them, in order to find the coffin of Joseph.

When a child grows up in a family that is prejudiced against a certain person, that prejudice is almost irremovable. If Moses was raised in the house of Amram, and Amram was raised in the house of Kehat, and Kehat was raised in the house of Levi, Moses should have been prejudiced against Joseph. How is it that for forty years in the desert he kept the coffin of Joseph "*immo bi-mehitzato*, within his precinct" (*Pesahim* 67a)? He refused to entrust the coffin to anyone else. If the tradition of the Levites was so hostile to Joseph, why did Moses bother with Joseph at all?

Levi must have changed his mind about Joseph. Instead of hating him, he revised his view in the last years of his life because he realized who Joseph was. Apparently, Levi, like the rest of his brothers, reappraised Joseph's personality, and in the course of the years they spent in Egypt, he and they discovered the beauty, saintliness, and greatness of Joseph's personality. Moses as a child heard many beautiful stories about Joseph, about that handsome lad sold into slavery, about his charm and beauty, about his humility and kindness, his sacrificial life and his simplicity, and his great accomplishment for Jewish history—for Joseph paved the way of dignity and majesty for the Jew exiled from the Promised Land. Moses heard many stories about how Joseph showed that it is possible for the Jew to serve the Almighty in the midst of luxury and opulence, in the midst of an inimical environment, that it is ridiculous to fear that gigantic pyramids will eclipse the sunlight of Abraham's tradition. That was shown by Joseph, by no one else.

If Moses was so concerned that he carried Joseph's coffin on his shoulders for forty years, it means that Moses considered Joseph to be his master and teacher. "The wise in heart will heed commandments" (Pr. 10:8). Moses came to love him and to admire him. That is why he considered himself the guardian of Joseph's bones, the executor of his will. Joseph may have lost the monarchy, but he won Moses our teacher as a student.

❧ *At the Burning Bush*

Petuhah: *A New Phase in Jewish History*

The Torah records several stories about Moses' early life (Ex. chap. 2). First, we are told of his birth and the way he was saved from the Nile by Pharaoh's daughter, who adopted him, and by Miriam, who brought him back to his mother. Then we are told about Moses' killing an Egyptian who was striking a Jew, and then about his reprimanding a Jew who was beating a fellow Jew. Next, we hear about Moses' flight from Egypt and how he became the son-in-law of Jethro, the priest of Midian. Moses then fathered a son, whom he named Gershom.

After the Torah tells us that Zipporah gave birth to Gershom (Ex. 2:22), there is a *petuhah* in the Torah scroll, a blank space followed by a new paragraph or section. The new section begins:

> And it came to pass in the course of those many days, that the king of Egypt died; and the Children of Israel groaned by reason of their bondage, and they cried out, and their cry rose up to God by reason of their bondage (Ex. 2:23).

Why is there a *petuhah* before these verses?

The *petuhah* signifies that a new reality is about to emerge. The bondage in Egypt had been a time of *hester panim*, the hiding of God's face, a period when man feels completely alienated from God. During *hester panim*, man becomes like any other living organism, like a brute in the field or forest. He is no longer under the unique, individual protection of the Almighty. During the time of *hester panim*, the Jews' suffering becomes routine. Survivors of the Nazi concentration camps relate that after a time, they began to think their lives had to be like this, that it was useless to complain, ridiculous to cry, pointless to scream. *Hester panim* is a time of silence. But after "many days," they began to groan, and "God heard their groaning, and God remembered His covenant with Abraham, with Isaac, and with Jacob" (Ex. 2:24).

Suddenly, the period of *hester panim* was over: "And God looked upon the Children of Israel, *va-yeida E-lohim*, and God knew" (Ex. 2:25). The word "*va-yeida*" has multiple meanings. In our context, it conveys the idea that God shared, that He became involved, that He participated in the suffering of His people. This is the concept of *Shekhinta be-galuta*, the Divine Presence in exile. Until now, the people were strangers to Him; there was no involvement, but only complete estrangement and alienation. Yet after *yamim rabbim*, many dark, silent years, God became involved in the destiny of His people. That is why this section is presented as a new paragraph; it represents a new situation.

Once the Almighty turns his countenance toward His suffering people, day begins to dawn for them. The only thing missing is a redeemer. Therefore the next verse continues: "And Moses was tending the flock of Jethro his father-in-law, the priest of Midian . . ." (Ex. 3:1). The redeemer will be Moses.

A Reluctant Moses

Approximately sixty years elapsed between the time when Moses "was grown and he went out to his brothers" (Ex. 2:11) and the time when he returned to Egypt as an eighty-year-old man (see Ramban, Ex. 2:23). During those sixty years of *hester panim*, Moses was completely irrelevant to the Jewish people. There was no need for him.

It is therefore understandable that when the star of redemption began to rise and Moses had to take a leadership role, he was not ready. "Moses was tending the flock of Jethro his father-in-law, the priest of Midian" (Ex. 3:1).

Why do we care to whom the flock belongs? Moreover, we already know that Jethro is Moses' father-in-law, as we are told just a few verses earlier that Moses married Jethro's daughter Zipporah (2:21). Why does the Torah, which is so careful about even a single unnecessary letter, repeat Jethro's position?

The Torah is trying to portray Moses' complete alienation from his people. He was the son-in-law of Jethro, the priest of Midian, and enjoyed being a member of Midianite society. Moses was completely absorbed in his daily chores; he was completely integrated into the Midianite environment. He was part and parcel of Jethro's family. This is why the Torah emphasizes the fact that Jethro was Moses' father-in-law; there was a certain closeness, friendship, and love between them.

Moses forgot his past—not due to old age, but because he wanted to forget. Moses purposely dismissed from his mind all the memories of his youth, of leaving the royal palace and going out to his brethren with the honest and sincere intention of helping them. Moses was alienated from his people; he simply wanted to extinguish his memories because of his bitter and tragic experience with the people in Egypt.

Earlier, Moses had possessed the ambition to be a leader. He was a royal prince, raised to be the successor to Pharaoh. Yet he somehow identified with the people whom the Egyptians viewed with disdain and contempt. Moses wanted to join them, to identify with those subhumans, the oppressed and tortured slaves. But when he reprimands one Israelite for striking another, he is rebuked in a horrible way: "Who made you a prince and judge over us? Do you intend to kill me, as you killed the Egyptian?" (Ex. 2:14). So he forgot them. He made himself a Midianite.

Indeed, in his attempt to distance himself from his people, he *intentionally* forgot them. We know that a person can make himself forget, as in the case of Pharaoh's chief butler: "Nevertheless the chief butler did not remember Joseph, but forgot him" (Gen. 40:23)—he forgot him because he *wanted* to forget him. Why should he remember the time that he spent in jail together with some unknown Hebrew? Moses similarly tried to forget his past and to become a shepherd in Midian.

Rashi quotes a *midrash* that sheds light on Moses' mentality. According to the midrashic interpretation, the incident of the two feuding Jews depressed Moses to such a degree that he gave up hope that the redemption would ever come: " 'Moses was frightened' (Ex. 2:14)—When he saw that among Israel there were wicked informers, he said: Perhaps now they are unworthy of redemption." Rashi continues: " '[Moses said:] Indeed, the matter is known' (Ex. 2:14)—The matter I was wondering about is now known: what sin did Israel, alone among the seventy nations, commit so as to be worthy of hard labor? But now I see that they were deserving of it." Moses was afraid, Rashi explains, because he believed that there was no hope for the slaves. He was concerned that they had stooped so low, that they had sunk so deeply in the abyss of degradation and inhumanity, that they would never be deserving of freedom and redemption. "Indeed, the matter is known"—their destiny is known. Moses began to believe that the Egyptians were to some extent right. The Jew is a slave because he does not deserve to be a master.

Moses was wrestling with a tremendous problem: Why were the Jews enslaved in such a cruel and ruthless way? Why were the Jews less deserving than any other nation? Now Moses thought he understood: they were informers! There was no devotion to one another; they lacked commitment. After all, Moses had killed an Egyptian in order to defend a Hebrew—no one else would have done it. He could do it only because he was a member of the royal family, and the Jews went and informed the authorities! Such a people did not deserve salvation and the help of God.

Moses' attitude may seem strange, but it apparently was overpowering; the experience cast a fierce spell upon him. Moses left Egypt with no hope and a broken spirit. The dark night of slavery would continue forever. There is no hope for such a people. Moses thought that the centuries-long slavery had left its mark; it had corrupted the people. They had lost their dignity, thereby forfeiting their claim and their right to be a covenantal community. The Torah conceals Moses' thoughts and tells us only that "he fled from Pharaoh" (Ex. 2:15), but he really ran from his own brethren as well. He fled Egypt discouraged, disenchanted, and in despair. He wanted to be the leader, but his offer was disdainfully rejected. It is understandable that he felt complete alienation from the people. Because Moses was alienated from his brethren, the Torah mentions Jethro and repeats that he was Moses' father-in-law.

God was ready to act, but there was no Moses. There were two reasons for Moses' absence. First, the potential leader whom providence had selected for this historic role was humble; he did not believe that he could be more than a shepherd. Moreover, he had fled Egypt and had parted from his brethren with the intention of never returning; he had no intention of renewing the kinship or the friendship or the common destiny that bound him to his brothers. "And he led the flock far away into the desert" (Ex. 3:1)—he wanted to get farther and farther away, away from thoughts about Egypt, away from his brethren and their suffering. As long as Moses was just a shepherd for Jethro, the redemption could not take place.

But at the very moment when God turned His face and became involved in the destiny of Moses' people, we find Moses changing from a shepherd into a redeemer.

Chasing a Lamb

What changed Moses' attitude? "And he led the flock far away into the desert, and he came to the mountain of God, to Horeb" (Ex. 3:1). The Midrash (Ex. Rabbah 2:2) asks a simple question: Why did he lead the flock so far into the wilderness? What attracted Moses? Onkelos was apparently also concerned with this question; he translates the verse as *"ve-dabar yat ana la-atar shefar re'aya"*—Moses was looking for good pastureland where he could graze his flock for a long time. The problem is that the area of Mount Sinai was called *horev* for a reason: it is arid and dry, hardly good land for pasture. The Midrash tells us a different story. A little lamb ran away from the flock and Moses pursued it. Ordinarily, Moses, the experienced shepherd, would have caught up with it in a short time. A lamb is not a gazelle! But this time, something unusual happened—the lamb ran a like a deer. Moses could not keep pace with her. She ran, he ran; he could not catch her. So he kept pursuing the lamb until the lamb stopped at a spring and drank from its water.

This is not simply a nice story about a lamb, but a profound one about a person. The lamb symbolizes Moses; Moses ran from and after himself. Moses was the master of prophets, the future redeemer, and the greatest of all teachers. But there was a part of him that was hidden, unknown even to himself. There was a part of him that, like the lamb, rebelled somehow. Moses himself was not acquainted with that Moses, just as we are often not truly acquainted with ourselves. I may know my neighbors and friends well, but I don't know myself. Moses knew himself as a Midianite, completely alienated from his brethren, completely unconcerned with their destiny and future, but this little lamb began to run. Moses rebelled. He fled from the flock. He is the lamb that ran at a dizzying speed away from his persona as "Moses the son-in-law of Jethro," away from the Midianite establishment, away from the Moses who tried hard to forget the past, who tried not to think of his brethren who had lost their dignity and were doomed to eternal slavery and degradation. The lamb was Moses the restless and rebel-lious, Moses the dreamer, Moses the visionary, the young Moses who had been hidden within the new Moses for decades. Moses the searcher ran away from the practical, sedate, logical, realis-tic Moses, the son-in-law of Jethro.

The unknown Moses was thirsty. Apparently, the water that Moses had stored up in Midian and taken along with him into the wilderness could not quench the thirst of the other Moses, who ran off to look for a spring. Moses was running toward a spring whose whereabouts he himself did not know.

There is a beautiful story told by R. Nahman of Breslov about a heart and a spring. There is a heart, the central organ, which gives the heartbeat to the world. The world also has a spring, but the heart has never seen it. The heart is questing, pursuing the spring. From time to time, it catches an almost inaudible sound, the soft murmur of the flowing waters. This is how R. Nahman of Breslov portrayed man's quest for God. You can't see Him, but you quest for Him. You hear something—the flowing waters.

Moses heard the murmur of the flowing waters, the soft, almost inaudible sound that guided him toward the spring. But the lamb was too parched; the stored-up water could not quench its burning thirst. The lamb continued to run to a new source of water; the lamb ran and Moses the unknown ran.

Moses of the establishment was suddenly confronted with an unusual scene. First, he found a spring whose waters quenched his thirst, and then he saw the burning bush. This is where the change took place. The eighty-year-old Moses the capable shepherd of his father-in-law Jethro who had tried to erase from his memory all links with his brethren and to termi-nate all responsibility for their destiny—was defeated by anoth-er Moses. The young lad, the visionary Moses, overpowered his older self.

Some people lose their inner child as they mature. They stop dreaming and hoping and become very practical, pragmatic, and utilitarian. But in some people, no matter how mature they are, a little boy remains. From time to time, the old man some-how retraces his steps and turns into a little boy, a dreamer with imagination, who searches around the corner for a miracle.

The Midrash describes the contest between Moses, the mature man with the great intellect, who was practical and log-ical, and who saw no hope for his brethren, and the Moses of sixty years before, who shed his princely garments and went out among his brothers in order to become the redeemer. Back then, he believed in that mission. This was a race between the lamb, Moses as a young visionary, and the old, realistic, practical Moses. And the lamb won. By the time Moses caught up to the lamb, he could no longer go on being just Jethro's son-in-law, because it was then that he saw the burning bush.

"And he came to the mountain of God, to Horeb"—why is it called "the mountain of God"? Rashi (Ex. 3:1) explains, "It is so called because of future events," because the Torah was to be given on Mount Sinai. But why was this mountain chosen for the giving of the Torah? We all know, of course, the story that *Hazal* recount regarding Sinai's humility compared to other mountains. But I believe the answer is that Mount Sinai was chosen because something happened there before the Torah was given—Moses' victory over himself. At that spot, the young lad defeated the old man in Moses. It was there that Moses found himself.

Kierkegaard said, and I fully agree, that at the very moment a man finds himself, he finds God. At the burning bush, Moses found himself, and he thus found God. That is why the moun-tain is called here "the mountain of God." When God wanted to select a mountain for the public revelation, He selected Mount Sinai, because the first confrontation, the first rendezvous between God and man, had already taken place there.

The mountain was named "the mountain of God" at the very instant that Moses, exhausted from the race with the lamb, with himself, arrived at the spring and gave the triumphant lamb something to drink. The rendezvous between God and the individual is as significant as the meeting between God and six hundred thousand people.

The Message of the Malakh Hashem

When the Holy One is ready to do something, to realize a vision, to punish or to reward, He sends someone as his messenger. He very seldom sends an angel; He usually sends a human being with great personal qualities to fulfill the mission. But before Moses can be sent, he must change his opinion about the people; he must be ready to accept the assignment. Moses must change himself from an obscure shepherd in Midian into the great leader and the redeemer of Israel. This is why God spends so much time persuading Moses, without issuing commands. He wanted Moses to understand on his own the importance of redemption and the possibility of its occurring. The Midrash says that God spoke to Moses for seven days, and Moses only gave in on the last day (Ex. Rabbah 3:14). When Moses finally said that he was prepared to go, the redemption began.

When the Torah speaks of the revelation of a *malakh*, an angel, it sometimes uses the term *malakh E-lohim*, while at other times, the Torah uses the substitute *malakh Hashem*. The name *E-lohim* represents that God is the *ba'al ha-kohot*, the source of the unlimited dynamics of the cosmos and the natural law that prevails everywhere. The opening *parashah* of the Torah, which describes the creation of the world, begins "*Bereishit bara E-lohim*"—*E-lohim* is the Creator, the Architect, the Engineer, the all-powerful God. A *malakh E-lohim* is sent to exercise power, to intervene in the cosmic order.

In our context, a *malakh Hashem* appears in the fire of the burning bush (Ex. 3:2), but it would seem that a *malakh E-lohim* would have been appropriate here. The entire purpose of the rendezvous between Moses and the *malakh* was the announcement that God would intervene in the cosmic process in order to take the people out of Egypt. Why was a *malakh Hashem* used instead?

The purpose of the *malakh* was to give a message to Moses. While it is true that God told him that, if necessary, He would intervene to make the Egyptians send the Jews away, this was not the main purpose of the message. God wanted to reassure Moses, not so much regarding his ability, but regarding the people's worthiness of freedom.

"*Ra'oh ra'iti et oni ammi*—I have surely seen the affliction of My people that is in Egypt" (Ex. 3:7). The Midrash asks why the phrase "*ra'oh ra'iti,* I have surely seen," is used, when "*ra'iti,* I have seen," would have been sufficient. The Midrash answers beautifully, "*Moshe, attah ro'eh re'iyah ahat, va-ani ro'eh shetei re'iyot*"—you see the people only from one viewpoint, and I see the people from multiple viewpoints (Ex. Rabbah 3:1). You see the people simply as primitive pagans who, because of slavery and oppression and misery, are not the successors of the mission that Abraham tried to pass on to his children. They are not *My* people. However, I see two things. It is true that from time to time they may stoop very low. They may fall. But these people have the tremendous ability to rise suddenly. Your estimation of your people is wrong. As a human being, you see only the surface; your glance cannot penetrate into the innermost essence of My people. "*Ra'oh ra'iti*"—I can see from a multiple viewpoint the pain and the distress of "*ammi*, My people." You gave up on them; I did not. When you encountered the two feuding Jews and were the target of informers, you gave up and ran away and assimilated yourself into the Midianite community. But I have not given up. The word *am* is a derivative of *im*; they are My people, and I am with them.

You condemned the people because one individual acted wrongly toward you. You still remember that episode after sixty years, and it is time to forget it. You are wrong in your estimation of the people. They are not bad, although the surface, the exterior, may sometimes look that way. It is true that sometimes they do not display the proper dignity that I expect of the children of Abraham, Isaac, and Jacob. But deep down in their personalities, they are still the chosen people. Sometimes the exterior and the interior contradict each other. Sometimes the Jew acts wrongly, but this does not desecrate his personality as such.

Moses could not penetrate into the depths, into the hidden recesses of their personalities, and that is why he condemned them. But God looked at them with both eyes—"*ra'oh ra'iti*"—and He determined that they were ready for redemption.

God saw not the external personality of the Jews, but the deep part of their personality. You see contemptible slaves who only want to be on friendly terms with the taskmaster and the officer in order to gain a bigger portion of meat. You see the contemptible bondman in them, but you do not see the member of a kingdom of priests and a holy nation.

"*Et oni ammi asher be-Mitzrayim*"—they are still *be-Mitzrayim*, in slavery, and that is why you do not see them properly. You cannot expect a person who is exposed to torture and humiliation and suffering day in and day out, whose children are snatched away from the arms of their mother, who must always complete a quota of bricks lest he be beaten by the taskmaster—you cannot expect him to be a prophet, an aristocrat of the spirit, a priest, a king, or a great personality. You, Moses, see "*asher be-Mitzrayim*," and, yes, Egypt is filthy and contemptible. But "*ra'oh ra'iti*"—I see "*oni ammi*, the affliction of My people." I see their tragedy, their inability to be, at this juncture, what I want them to be. But they are capable of being "My people"; they are not yet "My people" because, alas, they are the nation "that is in Egypt."

"*Ra'oh ra'iti*" represents the finest idea in Judaism. These two words that God addressed to Moses when he began his assignment are what make repentance possible. All our hopes and aspirations for the arrival of the Messiah are based on these two words, on our belief that God sees past the filth and into the recesses of our souls.

God saw their pain before the nation itself realized it. Sometimes, if a person finds himself in distress, a close friend or relative will realize the danger and the risk before the person himself has a chance to understand. They only started moaning and groaning after Pharaoh died, when their lives became unbearable. But God heard their cries even before they started to complain, even during the dark night of silent slavery.

That was the main message that God wanted Moses to receive. For such a message, one does not send a *malakh E-lohim*. A *malakh E-lohim* comes with lightning and thunder, with plagues like blood and frogs, lice and pestilence. Here, God wished to give a message of hope and consolation to the people through Moses, at the same time that he reprimanded Moses for his skeptical approach to the people, for his losing faith in them. God wished to proclaim those dirty, unworthy slaves as *"ammi,"* members of My people. For that, He sent not a *malakh E-lohim*, but a *malakh Hashem*.

At the burning bush, God proclaims that He will protect His people because they are worthy of protection. Moses, said God, you are making a mistake. You gave up on them, but you are wrong. The *malakh Hashem* protects them; their identity will be preserved and they will not be assimilated into Egyptian society. The silent period, the period of anonymity when the Jew could not complain, would come to an end, and the Jew would emerge victorious. "And *malakh Hashem* appeared to him in the flame of fire out of the midst of the bush"—they will survive because of the *malakh Hashem*.

The Bush Was Not Consumed

Rashi (Ex. 3:2) cites and abridges the *midrash*: Why did God appear from the midst of a bush and not some other tree? Why did God choose to give His revelation in a primitive plant?

"Because 'I am with him in distress' (Ps. 91:15)." I share their travail; I am with them in times of crisis. When Israel experiences life as if it were a thorny bush, when Israel lives a degraded, foul life, I am with her; I share her pain.

There are many attributes of God: "merciful and gracious, long-suffering and abundant in love and truth," and so on (Ex. 34:6). In our text we see God as the *"shokheni seneh*, He who dwelt in the bush," as Moses later referred to Him in his blessing to the tribe of Joseph: "For the goodwill of He who dwelt in the bush, *u-retzon shokheni seneh*, let the blessing come upon the head of Joseph" (Deut. 33:16). The fact that God dwelt in a thornbush becomes an attribute of the Almighty, and He exhibits *ratzon*, in the sense of love (as in *ahavah ve-ratzon*).

When man encounters disaster, God is *immo*; His presence rises up. "Then the Lord answered Job out of the whirlwind" (Job 38:1). Even when a man finds himself in the depths of disaster and tragedy, even when he has lost everything and is completely lonely, stripped of everything that he had, God does not desert him. All individuals experience darkness at some point, finding themselves in the whirlwind of unexpected troubles. God resides even in that whirlwind. Job kept asking questions, even though the proper way out of his suffering was to praise God and to promote goodwill on the part of the Almighty. When Job finally admitted fault and stopped inquiring as to the metaphysics of evil, "the Lord gave Job twice as much as he had before" (Job 42:10). This is *shokheni seneh*, God who resides in the thornbush.

God's presence is the *Shekhinah*, and it is with man not only during physical distress but in spiritual distress as well. Even when a person has been involved in sin, God never deserts him. He is in the thornbush even though it is coarse, even though it bears no fruit and has no beauty, and even though all it can cause is pain. God is right there in the middle. Thus, when man knows how to address himself to God, he receives a response immediately.

"And he looked, and behold, the bush burned with fire, but the bush was not consumed" (Ex. 3:2). The simple understanding is that, although the thornbush was on fire, it never turned into ashes. There can also be a different interpretation. The angel appeared to Moses "in the flame of fire out of the midst of the bush." Imagine the bush as a geometric circle, and the fire as a concentric circle in the center of the bush. The angel was *be-labbat esh*, which Rashi translates as "in the heart of the fire," in the center of the inner circle. In other words, the fire was in the center and did not pass to the periphery. The flame was isolated somehow; it contained itself.

There were actually two miracles here. First, the bush was indestructible: "The bush burned with fire, but the bush was not consumed." This is what caught Moses' attention at first. But when Moses notes the miracle, he says, "I will turn now aside and see this great sight, why the bush is not burnt"—he was not impressed by the fact the bush was not *consumed*, but rather by the fact that the fire did not spread to the bush and was contained within the bush's center.

Why was Moses more impressed by the second miracle than the first? The two miracles symbolize two different things. The first showed that, no matter how difficult the circumstances or how great the suffering, the Jewish people—the covenantal community—is indestructible: "the bush was not consumed." We will never be consumed by fire or by the winds of time, because we are an eternal people. If we did not believe in this principle, we would stop building schools and stop trying to influence the modern Jew to commit himself to our covenantal tradition.

The second miracle expresses something different, *ra'oh ra'iti*: a Jew's external personality is not always indicative of his inner commitment. There is sometimes a conflict between the Jew's external and inner personalities, but regardless of the outside, deep down in his heart there is warm sensitivity and love. In the center of his heart, in the depths of his personality, there is a fire burning, and a Jew should never be expelled from or considered worthless to the Jewish community.

This message was crucial not only for Moses thousands of years ago, but is so for us as well. No Jew should be given up on as hopeless! A Jew may look quite like a thornbush, very scratchy, vulgar, hurtful, and insensitive. We might think that it does not pay to concern ourselves with him. But in truth we must try to expand our concern to embrace everyone.

My grandfather R. Hayyim did not exclude a single Jew, and because he did not expel or excommunicate, because he spoke to Jews as they passed by, he influenced many. If Moses had excommunicated the Jews in Egypt, what would have happened to us? We dare not resent nonobservance; we must have faith in the Jew, and must have hope that no matter how far he has removed himself from the traditional community, there is some fire within his personality. Sometimes it is nearly invisible, and only a Moses can see it, but it is there if you look for it.

Moses was interested in the second miracle more than the first. Moses was still confident that outside forces could not destroy the Jewish community. But Moses was the son of Amram, the son of Kehat; his great-grandfather was Levi, and his family led a sacrificial life, teaching the people how to perpetuate the covenantal tradition. And Moses saw that the Jew could violate this commitment. Because of his unpleasant experience with cynicism, with the readiness to inform, Moses doubted whether the Jewish way of life and identity still existed. Moses knew that we can resist external forces, but if the fire is out and the Jews have lost their Jewish identity, then the situation is hopeless. That was the problem that interested Moses; that is what instigated him to say, "I will turn now aside and see this great sight, why the bush is not burnt." Why is the fire not visible on the outside? Is it possible for a fire to be hidden? Apparently, he learned, it is possible for a person to hide a spiritual fire. In that case, the religious state of my brothers should no longer discourage me.

Many Jews have themselves forgotten about this inner flame. They consider themselves too far gone; they think that they cannot return on the road leading back to the Almighty. These Jews do not know that deep down within the recesses of their personalities the fire still burns, even if their outside is cold, dreary, sad, and obnoxious. Every person hates himself at certain times. This happens because we do not know about the flame in the center of the bush. We do not like what we see in the mirror, but if that mirror could reflect more than our faces, if it could show our spiritual personalities, we would discover a pleasant surprise—we are much better looking than we think we are.

Rashi makes a strange comment on the verse "I will turn now aside and see this great sight"—"I will turn away from here to come close to there." What does Rashi add to the verse? He is explaining that the verse is not talking about geographic space. Moses was not turning aside from a physical position; he was turning aside from his previous worldview and embracing a new outlook, a new philosophy on life. Let me turn aside, he is saying, from the categories which I used to use. I will adopt other categories, other concepts, other ideas.

Moses was also intrigued by the fact that God, who was in the center of the burning bush, did not "spread." God could have revealed Himself in thunder and lightning; He could have spoken from infinity, from transcendence. Instead, God spoke to Moses from no place at all, from the center of a circle. The One who cannot be confined by the heavens can yet confine Himself to a thornbush. Moses told the tribe of Joseph: Satisfy the will not only of the *shokhen Marom* (Is. 33:5), the God who dwells on high, but also of "He who dwelt in the bush." This self-contraction represents humility and modesty.

When Moses realized the messages of the burning bush—God's identification with His people, the flame within every Jew, and God's *middat ha-tzimtzum*, His ability to contract Himself in our world, God told the *malakh* that he was no longer necessary. That is how Moses was appointed the redeemer.

Hashem *Replaces* E-lohim

The moment Moses turned away from Jethro's flock in order to see the bush, he precipitated two changes. First, the angel disappeared; God Himself was now residing in the bush and spoke to him from there. A *malakh* is a messenger, a plenipotentiary, but we have a rule that *mitzvah bo yoter mi-bi-sheluho*: a messenger may perform his job well, but it is always preferable that the individual himself do it (*Kiddushin* 41a). The Jews were now under the supervision and protection not of an angel, but of the Almighty Himself.

But there is a second change as well—"And *Hashem* saw that he turned aside to see" (Ex. 3:4). Earlier, the name *E-lohim* was used, but now the Tetragrammaton appears. "And it came to pass in the course of those many days . . . they cried out, and their cry rose up to *E-lohim* by reason of the bondage. And *E-lohim* heard their cry . . . And *E-lohim* looked upon the Children of Israel, and *E-lohim* knew" (Ex. 2:23–25). The name *Hashem* does not appear in that previous chapter. When God suffered with them, when He shared in their distress, He was *E-lohim*. But they still had to wait for redemption; *Hashem* was not there yet. Only when Moses said, "*Asura na ve-er'eh*, I will turn now aside and see," do we read, "*Va-yar Hashem*, And *Hashem* saw." The time of the redemption has arrived.

God later told Moses that he had been singled out as the chosen prophet, the father of all future prophets. He was different from everyone else. "And I appeared to Abraham, Isaac, and Jacob, by the name of *E-l Sha-dai*, but by My name *Hashem* I was not known to them" (Ex. 6:3). God did not make His explicit name available to them, but it is at Moses' disposal.

E-l Sha-dai and *E-lohim* represent promises and the ability to wait. Abraham waited, Isaac waited, Jacob waited. God told Abraham of four hundred years of exile: "Your seed shall be a stranger in a land that is not theirs, and shall serve them, and they shall afflict them for four hundred years" (Gen. 15:13). The use of the names *E-lohim* and *E-l Sha-dai* indicates that, even though Israel is protected during the era of silence and suffering, God has not yet kept His word: "I have promised but not yet fulfilled" (Rashi, Ex. 6:3).

When Moses came complaining, "Why have You dealt ill with this people? Why have You sent me? For since I have come to Pharaoh to speak in Your name, he has done evil to this people; and neither have You delivered Your people at all" (Ex. 5:22), God lamented the absence of the patriarchs. Rashi (Ex. 6:9), based on the Gemara (*Sanhedrin* 111a), quotes God as rebuking Moses: How lamentable is it that Abraham, Isaac, and Jacob are gone! I revealed Myself to them many times, and they did not ask for My name. I promised Abraham the whole Land of Israel, and yet when he came to bury Sarah, he had to buy a grave and was overcharged. Isaac dug wells, and the wells were taken away. I gave Jacob the land, and then, when he came back to Shechem, he had to buy a plot of land. Yet they never complained; they never had doubts as to My truthfulness and My ability to fulfill My promises.

E-lohim refers to God who requires that a Jew have faith, patience, and perseverance. It is very hard to wait. And yet the Jew waits and waits. Every day, he says the *Ani Ma'amin*—I believe in the coming of the Messiah, and even though he may tarry I will wait for him every day. The Jew who communicates with *E-lohim*, then, is greater than the Jew who communicates with *Hashem*, the fulfiller of promises. When God bestows grace upon the people, it is not so difficult to be a Jew. Nevertheless, during the long, lonely night of exile, the Jew did not lose his faith in *E-lohim*; *Hashem* did not reveal Himself. The Jew who waits is great indeed.

When Moses said, "I will turn aside now and see," *Hashem* appeared; the time to fulfill promises was at hand. The redemption began not on the first night of Pesah, when the actual

Exodus took place, but when Moses was confronted by God, even before he was convinced to accept his calling.

The Great Sight

Moses referred to the strange sight of the burning bush as *"ha-mar'eh ha-gadol ha-zeh*, this great sight." It would seem to have been more appropriate to refer to it as a *nes* or a *pele*, a miracle or a wonder. Why does he stress that it is "great"? Apparently, Moses was intrigued not by the miraculous nature of the event, but by its greatness. It is not always necessary for an event to be miraculous in order to be great, and not every miraculous event is a great event.

A unique event might not have any real significance. A "great" event, on the other hand, is an event that changes a person or ushers in a new era; it is great in its results, regardless of whether it was supernatural. Moses recognized that this was not just a strange fire, a phenomenon that had to be investigated. He immediately attributed great significance to it—it was a *mar'eh gadol*. Moses felt this intuitively, before God revealed anything to him; his accelerated heartbeat told him that something great was happening, something for which he had waited.

A wasted event is a small event, even if it is miraculous. *Hazal* downplayed miracles and insisted that a person should not expect or rely upon a miracle occurring for him (*Pesahim* 64b and *Yerushalmi Shekalim* 6:3). But we do appreciate the greatness precipitated by the miracle. We appreciate man's interpretation of a miracle and man's ability to turn a miracle into a great, creative event. The Talmud tells us that the festival of Hanukkah was established only after a full year had passed after the miracle of the oil that burned for eight days (*Shabbat* 21a). Why did they wait a full year? Why did they not immediately establish a holiday? Because the miracle per se is not deserving of a new holiday. *Hazal* waited to see how the Jews benefited from the miracle; would it become a great event, or would it remain a small event? They wanted to study the results of the miracle—did the people understand the meaning of the event, had they taken advantage of the opportunities that were offered to them by the event? If the miracle had not been understood by the crowd, and life had remained just as dreary and meaningless after the miracle as before, the festival of Hanukkah would never have come into existence. After a year, the Sages of that period realized that the miracle had accomplished a great deal. The community had developed a new outlook on life.

Moses saw *"ha-mar'eh ha-gadol ha-zeh"*; he saw great potential for a change in Jewish destiny. The Exodus is a result of that encounter of Moses with the Almighty.

"Moses Moses"

After God saw that Moses had turned aside, "God called out to him from amid the bush and said, 'Moses Moses,' and he replied, 'Here I am' " (Ex. 3:4). God calls out to Moses by repeating his name: *Moses, Moses*. This phenomenon is seen elsewhere in the Bible. God summoned, *"Abraham, Abraham"* (Gen. 22:11). He called out, *"Jacob, Jacob"* (Gen. 46:2). He called, *"Samuel, Samuel"* (I Sam. 3:10). (Samuel was the only one who did not immediately respond "Here I am," because he did not realize who was calling him.) But there is a difference between "Moses Moses" and the other name repetitions. In all the other instances, there is a *pesik*, a line indicating a pause, between the names—"Abraham, *pesik*, Abraham"; "Jacob, *pesik*, Jacob." In the case of Moses, however, there is no pause.

When God addressed Himself to Abraham, He called out, "Abraham," and He paused. When Abraham did not answer, He said "Abraham" a second time. God waited, perhaps for a fraction of a second. The same is true of Jacob. But when He called out to Moses, there was no pause; He said "Moses Moses" in one breath, as it were.

Why is Moses different? There is no reason to assume that he responded more quickly than Abraham and Jacob, for at the beginning of his career, Moses was completely inexperienced at prophecy. I think that "Moses Moses" is, rather, an expression of urgency. If there is a fire in your house and your son is sleeping upstairs, you will likely cry out, "Moses, Moses, Moses!" You would repeat his name out of urgency, not because you are waiting for a response.

In the case of Moses, God was, so to speak, desperate. He tells Moses that if he accepts the mission, if he accepts the task of redeemer, everything will be all right; if not, everything will be wasted. There was a sense of urgency in the repetition of Moses' name.

Moses and Abraham

To continue our comparisons between Moses and the patriarchs, who was greater, Abraham or Moses? We are informed of Moses' greatness in *Parashat Beha'alotekha*. Miriam asked, "Has the Lord indeed spoken only with Moses? Has He not spoken also with us?" (Num. 12:2). God responded that not only was Moses a greater prophet than she; Moses was qualitatively different— "Not so My servant Moses; he is trusted in all My house; with him do I speak mouth to mouth" (Num. 12:7–8). In this regard, Moses is above even Abraham, Isaac, and Jacob.

When did Moses achieve this exalted position as the greatest prophet? After Moses ascended Mount Sinai the first time to receive the tablets, the Torah does not describe Moses at all. The second time, however, we are told that his face began to radiate or generate light (Ex. 34:29). It was then that Moses was established as the father of the prophets.

Until that point, the patriarchs were superior to Moses. But after the sin of the golden calf, Moses expressed his willingness to sacrifice himself for the sake of the people—"Erase me, I pray, from Your book which You have written" (Ex. 32:32). At that point, Moses was raised to a higher level and became the greatest of all prophets, both those before and those after him. No other prophet was entrusted with the Torah. Not even

Abraham, Isaac, and Jacob could have given a mitzvah to the people, and "No future prophet [after Moses] may innovate a law" (*Sifra, Behukkotai* 8:13).

If Moses was so great, why don't we refer in the *Amidah* to "the God of Moses," just as we refer to "the God of Abraham"? There is an inherent difference between Abraham and Moses. According to the Midrash, echoed by Maimonides (*Hilkhot Avodat Kokhavim* 1:3), Abraham searched for God, but God did not react immediately. It was only much later, after Abraham had come to believe in Him, that God told him, "Go forth from your land" (Gen. 12:1). Moses was just the opposite. Moses did not search for the Almighty. He was a shepherd for Jethro, and "he hid his face because he feared to look at God" (Ex. 3:6). God searched for Moses, and He found him. Abraham, Isaac, and Jacob are the only true forefathers; God's revelation to them came after a long time and many frustrated efforts.

Model for the Future Redemption

What theological principles about redemption can we derive from this story of God and Moses? First, we are duty-bound to believe that the people will eventually be redeemed, no matter how long it takes. This, as we saw above, is the principle expressed in the verse "And I appeared to Abraham, Isaac, and Jacob, by the name *E-l Sha-dai*, but by My name *Hashem* I was not known to them" (Ex. 6:3)—sometimes we must wait for God's promises to be fulfilled. We are a people whose identity was forged in suffering. No other nation in history has suffered as much as the Jewish people. We have survived because we are believers like Abraham; even though we experienced God as *E-l Sha-dai*, we have maintained our faith contrary to all logical arguments. The Jewish people have demonstrated tremendous patience and perseverance. We have been confronted by many obstacles and temptations, but we are still here.

Second, God sends a human being to arrange the redemption. The Holy One could have redeemed the people Himself, of course. He debated with Moses for seven days to convince him to accept this mission, because while God is the true Redeemer, He chooses a human to perform the physical aspect of redemption. In Egypt, Moses was the qualified messenger, and in the future, God will appoint a human being who meets all the qualifications to be the redeemer.

Moses objected to his mission. He felt that he was not qualified for his mission to speak to Pharaoh or to lead the Children of Israel out of Egypt. Aaron, who had been raised among his people, was far more qualified than he. God explains to Moses that he is the appropriate messenger: "This is the *ot* that I have sent you: when you have brought the people out of Egypt, you shall worship God upon this mountain" (Ex. 3:12). *Ot* here does not mean "sign," but "reason." This is the reason that I have chosen you, Moses, and no one else. If I wanted a great diplomat, orator, or organizer, I would have chosen Aaron or someone else. But I do not need all that; I can do that myself. What I need is a *melammed*, someone who will take slaves and, within seven weeks, convert them into "a kingdom of priests and a holy nation" who will worship Me on this mountain, someone who can teach them My commandments. For this job, Moses is supremely qualified. And this is exactly what the future King Messiah will do as well. He will possess the ability to teach Torah, to change a people, and to ennoble them and raise them to great heights.

Moses as Teacher [margin note]

❧ *Three Encounters*

Gaining Pharaoh's Respect

As the plagues leading up to the Exodus from Egypt draw to a close, the Torah tells us that "The man Moses was very great in the land of Egypt, in the sight of Pharaoh's servants, and in the sight of the people" (Ex. 11:3). It is very strange that Moses was so admired. After all, Egypt suffered much because of Moses, and its economy was ruined. Nevertheless, he was great in their eyes. Yet we read that just beforehand Moses and Aaron were summarily driven out—"*va-yegaresh otam*"—from Pharaoh's presence (Ex. 10:11). How can we account for that irreverent dismissal if he was so admired?

There are at least four answers that we can consider. The first is to be found in the observation of Rabbi Samson Raphael Hirsch (Ex. 11:2–3, s.v. *dabber na*) that it was only after the plague of darkness that Pharaoh and his people began to respect Moses. That was the critical moment, the turning point in the relationship of Moses with Pharaoh and the entire land of Egypt. In the history of wars we have not come across a situation where one party is completely enveloped in darkness and the second enjoys light. During the three dark days the Jews could have exterminated the population, plundered the land,

and departed from Egypt. The old Pharaoh had argued (Ex. 1:10) that if Egypt should get involved in a war, the Jews would support its enemy. The three days of darkness proved this charge to be completely false. Suddenly, Moses appeared as a charismatic leader, a great man who actually wanted to reform his people and liberate them from slavery. He became great in their eyes.

A second answer relies on the semantics of the word *va-yegaresh*, a legal term that does not mean physical removal of a person or simply telling them to get out; *va-yegaresh* connotes terminating a relationship, as when divorce is referred to as *gerushin*. Pharaoh suggested to Moses and Aaron that the males should go and the little ones remain in Egypt. Moses refused, and Pharaoh therefore cut off the negotiations. This does not suggest any lack of respect.

A third answer is that the dismissal by Pharaoh was actually feigned contempt. Pharaoh had to evict Moses and Aaron because he was afraid that his servants might give in if the argument were to continue. Pharaoh was a tyrant, a deity to his people—and yet his slaves had the arrogance to tell him, "Do you not know yet that Egypt is lost?" (Ex. 10:7). Are you ignorant of the fact that the land is in ruins? Why are you carrying on the conflict with them? Apparently, Moses had succeeded in convincing them, and Pharaoh thought that if he did not drive Moses out of his palace immediately, the servants might join Moses and demand the liberation of the Jews. Moses had made inroads into Pharaoh's entourage. Pharaoh had to dispose of all amenities and dismiss Moses because of the respect in which Moses was held by the Egyptians.

However, a fourth answer—and the best, I feel—is that Pharaoh was concerned not about his servants but about himself. He was entranced by Moses as much as his servants were; Moses fascinated him because of his personality. There is no other way to understand Pharaoh's tolerance. Moses had come into his palace to tell him to excuse the Jews from their work so that they might leave the country, and he threatened plagues if his demands were not met. Such a person should be either locked up or executed. Pharaoh's tolerance is one of the greatest miracles in the story of the Exodus!

Yet Moses' personality was, in fact, out of the ordinary. His charisma was so great that Pharaoh could not dissipate the spell that Moses' personality had cast upon him. That was what made Pharaoh tolerate Moses, regardless of the harm inflicted upon the Egyptian economy. Pharaoh was afraid that if his argument with Moses were to continue, he would yield to Moses' will. He felt Moses' charm immobilizing his mind, encroaching upon him. So he quickly dismissed him.

Let us recall Pharaoh's reaction when Moses and Aaron originally came to demand that the people be set free, at least for three days, so that they would have the opportunity to hold a feast to their God (Ex. 5:1–5). First of all, said Pharaoh, I do not know this God; why should I agree? Second, why do you interfere with the people's performance of their duty? Why do you disturb them and prevent their work? You, too, have some assignments, so go and attend to them. Pharaoh did not take seriously these two old men who were interfering with the work of the people. At the beginning of his encounter with Moses, Pharaoh was quite frank in stating that he was interested in preserving the prevailing social order. There was no reason for him to give up the source of income provided by the slaves.

At first, Pharaoh did not believe that Moses was truly concerned with worship and celebrating a feast in the desert. He thought that Moses either was not to be taken seriously or wanted the people to leave Egypt and never come back. He suspected Moses of planning to establish a kingdom of his own, of wanting the slaves to serve him and his cohort.

Later, Pharaoh understood that Moses and Aaron could not be ignored. He no longer had the contemptuous approach that the Torah depicts at the beginning of their encounter. He understood that Moses really intended to organize a community of committed people and to formulate a new code of morality. He began to understand that when they spoke about the feast in the wilderness, what they had in mind was something serious, namely, receiving the Torah. Pharaoh did not know exactly what it was, but he felt that it was something true and frighteningly mysterious. He therefore came up with a new approach: "See that evil (*ra'ah*) is before you" (Ex. 10:10). Pharaoh began to warn Moses not to embark on his proposed adventure. As Rashi (s.v. *re'u*) quotes him, Pharaoh says: I am an astrologer and I can foresee the future. There is a certain star which is rising to greet and usher you into history; this star will become your lode-star and its name is *ra*, which means disaster, catastrophe, and massacre.

Pharaoh warned Moses and Aaron that their people would arouse the hatred of the entire world because they would be looked upon as arrogant, proud, vain, and intolerant. The committed community would be treated as strangers in every land, regardless of the span of time they might spend there as citizens. The star of *ra* will trail you, he warned; destruction will follow your history. You will have to give in, to surrender and compromise. Pharaoh tells Moses to go without the children (Ex. 10:11). If the adults want to start such a community, they are entitled. They know their fate, and they are ready to take the risk of being hated by everybody. But by what right do you take the children along?

Pharaoh is not cynical any more; he does not ridicule Moses but argues with him at the moral level, telling him that he has no right to involve the little ones. As the king of Egypt, he cannot commit the crime of neglecting the safety of the children. He then quickly throws Moses out because he did not want to hear his answer. He was afraid that Moses might convince him.

A great man has an impact upon everybody he meets, and Moses had that impact not only upon Pharaoh, but upon all the members of Pharaoh's administration and the whole population of Egypt. Moses was chosen by the Holy One to transform a nation of slaves into a holy nation of priests. Liberating the people politically could have been done by anybody sent by the Almighty. But changing the slave mentality into that of a spiritual aristocrat could be done only by one man, Moses, the greatest teacher of all.

Leaving Egypt with Riches

When the Holy One met Moses for the first time, He charged him with the mission of going to Egypt and liberating the Jewish people. He did not tell him specifically how to accomplish this mission. Yet He did disclose to him a strange detail:

> I will give this people favor in the sight of Egypt; and it shall come to pass that when you go, you shall not go empty. Each woman shall request (*sha'alah*) of her neighbor, and from her that lived in her house, silver vessels and gold vessels, and garments, and you shall put them on your sons and daughters (Ex. 3:21–22).

Why was it necessary to inform Moses of this one detail at the very beginning? Indeed, the point is repeated later on:

> And the Lord said to Moses, Yet I will bring one plague more upon Pharaoh and upon Egypt; afterwards he will let you go from here. When he shall let you go, he shall surely thrust you out altogether from here. Speak now in the ears of the people, and let every man request (*ve-yish'alu*) of his neighbor, and every woman of her neighbor, silver vessels and gold vessels (Ex. 11:1–2).

Moreover, it is repeated yet a third time:

> And the children of Israel did according to the word of Moses and they requested (*va-yish'alu*) of Egypt silver vessels and gold vessels and garments. And the Lord

gave the people favor in the sight of Egypt, and they gave them what they requested (*va-yash'ilum*) (Ex. 12:35–36).

Why was this such an important feature in the story of the Exodus that it was repeated over and over?

When we read of the negotiations between Moses and Pharaoh, we get the impression that the Holy One did not want the Jews to liberate themselves, but rather wanted Pharaoh to finally agree to the liberation of the people. The Torah tells us that when a master liberates his Hebrew slave, his *eved Ivri*, he must "not let him go empty-handed" (Deut. 15:13). A gift is a sign of mutual respect and equality, and this must be acknowledged.

Interesting is the halakhah regarding giving the instrument of *kinyan* during a marriage (*Kiddushin* 7a; Maimonides, *Hilkhot Ishut* 5:22). Usually the groom gives the ring to the wife. However, what if the groom says "Behold, you are sanctified to me," but the ring is given by the woman to the man? True, the law requires that it be given by the man to the woman, but if the man is an important personality, an *adam hashuv*, there is no need to repeat the marriage ceremony. The mere fact that he accepted a gift from her is enough, because she derived so much pleasure from his accepting the ring that she consented to be married. When a very important person accepts a gift, the pleasure and satisfaction to the donor are of great value.

The Holy One wanted Pharaoh not only to liberate the Jews, but to see them as equals—and that was achieved. Moses was told to instruct the people: "Ve-yish'alu . . . silver vessels and gold vessels" (Ex. 11:2). *Yish'alu* does not mean "borrow"; it means "request." This explains why the Torah adds in the next verse, "And the Lord gave the people favor in the sight of Egypt; moreover, the man Moses was very great in the land of Egypt, in the sight of Pharaoh's servants, and in the sight of the people" (Ex. 11:3). Previously, Moses did not command respect from Pharaoh. By the end, he did. The Jews were respected, as confirmed by the fact that the people were eager to give them gifts, because the fact that the Jews accepted those gifts gave them pleasure and satisfaction. It means that the Jews were not liberated as inferior beings. At least for the final few days, they achieved the status of equals.

Suddenly they were liberated! But before long there would be a new request: "Speak to the Children of Israel that they bring Me an offering" for the *Mishkan*, the Tabernacle (Ex. 25:2). However, the Torah immediately instructs that the offering is not to be taken from every individual, but only "from every person whose heart so moves him" (ibid.). Everyone, poor and rich, must give the half-shekel, but the contribution to the Tabernacle is to be voluntary; no coercive means should be employed. The Romans considered *tzedakah* an act of charity, but the Torah considered it an act of justice. *Tzedakah* is an indebtedness; when we give charity to the poor, we pay our debt. Yet the Tabernacle was built only by those "whose heart stirred him up, and every one whom his spirit made willing" (Ex. 35:21).

We know how slaves are treated. They had no property, no valuable utensils, and no fine clothes. They saw the beautiful dresses on the Egyptian women while their children were in rags. They had been hungry, and suddenly they acquired wealth and opulence—the same clothes their masters had worn just weeks before. But soon after, there was an announcement: Contribute if you wish. There was no demand to give money, only a request, and they freely gave away to the Tabernacle all that they had gotten a few weeks before. They hallowed the Tabernacle with their ability to do what they knew was right without compulsion.

Amalek and Jethro

How should we interpret the continuity of the *parashiyot* which deal with the miracles that took place on the night of Pesah in Egypt (Ex. 11–13:16), the first stations at which the Jews camped in the desert (Ex. 13:17–17:7), and two stories—Jethro and Amalek—which at first glance appear completely out of context with the story of the Exodus (Ex. 17:8–18:27)?

The Book of Exodus did not have to tell us about Jethro's arrival, his reception by Moses, his advice about the judges, and his departure. These could have been related in the Book of Numbers, in *Beha'alotekha,* when Moses invited his father-in-law, "Come with us, and we will do good to you; for the Lord has spoken good concerning Israel" (Num. 10:29). However, the story of Jethro is placed in Exodus before that of *mattan Torah*, the giving of the Torah, and as soon as Jethro leaves, the Torah tells us—immediately, without a pause—that "In the third month . . . they entered the wilderness of Sinai . . . and there Israel camped before the mountain" (Ex. 19:1–2). Similarly, there is another non-Jew mentioned in the *parashiyot* that precede *mattan Torah*: Amalek. The Torah gives us a very precise report about the places where the Jews stopped, the places where they had water and did not have water, the story of the manna, and so forth. It then tells us the story of Amalek as if that episode, too, is indispensable to understand *mattan Torah*.

Apparently, before reading the story of *mattan Torah* (Ex. 19 ff.), we are supposed to know how Jethro was impressed by the events of the Exodus, how he decided to exchange paganism for Judaism, and how he went home determined to convert his household (as Rashi noted in his comment to Ex. 18:27). And, on the other hand, it is also important to know that Amalek was more excited than Jethro over what they heard, but that their conclusions were completely different. Amalek heard that there was a nation that could defy Egypt and gain freedom from Pharaoh, a nation guided by laws that were different from those prevailing throughout the world. Such a nation should not exist, Amalek concluded, and should be exterminated. Why is it important to know this before we hear the story of *mattan Torah*?

The Torah was given to Israel, to the covenantal community whose founders were Abraham, Isaac, and Jacob. However, the election of Israel to the exalted position of a holy nation has a universal aspect. Israel is charged with the mission of passing on the Torah and its morality to all of humanity. The Torah was given to us exclusively, but only for a limited time. When the messianic era begins, the Torah will be transmitted to mankind as a whole, and all will accept its teachings. The *Malkhuyot* section of the *Amidah* on Rosh Ha-Shanah is dedicated exclusively to that idea. We pray to God for this vision to be fulfilled and realized as soon as possible.

> *U-ve-khen ten pahdekha,* Instill Your awe upon all Your works, and Your dread upon all that You have created. Let all works revere You and all creatures prostrate themselves before You. Let them all become a single society. . . . And everyone who has breath in his nostrils will say, "The Lord, God of Israel, is King, and His kingship rules over all."

At Sinai, *mattan Torah* was an isolated event whose purpose was to confirm the covenant between the Almighty and the descendants of Abraham, Isaac, and Jacob. It was an intimate affair, a private wedding binding a single nation with the Holy One the way a covenant binds husband and wife. But *mattan Torah* was also an event of cosmic proportions, one that included not only six hundred thousand ex-slaves, but all of humanity, present and future. "The whole world trembled before You" (Rosh Ha-Shanah *Amidah*, *Shofarot*). There was not a single spot in the cosmos that was not aware that something unique and singular was transpiring. Not only human beings, but the beasts in the field—indeed, all living creatures—were involved in *mattan Torah*.

With the arrival of the Messiah and the beginning of the eschatological era, nature—which appears to us not only indifferent but hostile to our dreams, aspirations, and hopes—will also be redeemed. At present, there is no element of *hesed* in nature; it is complete *din*. When the world is redeemed by Torah, the element of *hesed* will be injected not only in the law guiding society, but in the cosmic behavior of nature. Moral law and the law of nature will merge. Isaiah prophesies, "The wolf shall dwell with the lamb" (Is. 11:6).

When Moses first ascended to Mount Sinai, the giving of the Torah was accompanied by thunder. The Holy One had to appear to His people in a way that would be audible to all humanity, resounding throughout the entire cosmos. It was necessary because all the peoples of the world had to know that this event would, in the end, have great significance for them and for the whole world. But when the second set of tablets was given, God told Moses, "And no man shall come up with you, neither let any man be seen throughout the entire mountain; neither let the flocks nor herds feed before the mountain" (Ex. 34:3). There was to be complete secrecy. Rashi (Ex. 34:3, s.v. *ve-ish*) explains: "Because the first tablets were given amidst great noises and alarms and a vast assembly, the evil eye had power over them; there is no finer quality than modesty." God told Moses: The world already knows, so I do not need any publicity this second time. Go up quietly.

Can the world eventually accept such a Torah? Is it morally and psychologically capable of forgoing many things that are pleasant and doing many things that are unpleasant? The vision of *mattan Torah* as a cosmic event that will eventually redeem everybody seemed to be undermined by Amalek's appearance as the archenemy of Israel.

Usually, the Torah mentions the event which motivated a certain individual to take action, either positive or negative. "Jethro heard about all that God had done for Israel" (Ex. 18:1) and decided to pay a visit to Moses. Balak saw the military might of Israel and invited Balaam to curse and destroy the people (Num. 22:2–5). Their actions were "rational." However, the

Torah simply tells us that "Amalek came and fought with Israel in Rephidim" (Ex. 17:8). What caused Amalek's arrival? Logically, Amalek had no reason to attack Israel.

A declaration of war is likely in four situations. First, there may be imperialistic interests. The king is an empire builder and therefore invades territories which belong to small, weak nations. However, Amalek was not motivated by imperialism, as the Jews had no territories to be occupied. "Remember what Amalek did to you while you were wandering" (Deut. 25:17). The Jews had nothing that could be taken from them.

Second, there might be fear that the opponent is planning a surprise attack. Sihon and Og came out to fight with the Jews because they wanted to prevent Israel from invading their countries. However, Amalek attacked the Jews when they were far away from Amalek's territory—"when you departed from Egypt," far away from Amalek.

Third, a war may break out because a government feels hurt. The people of one country might have inflicted damage or injury upon the citizens of a neighboring country and then refused to make amends. Amalek did not know the Jews; "They surprised you while you were on your way from Egypt" (Deut. 25:18). The Jews were surprised to be attacked by a strange, mysterious enemy.

Fourth, war may be designed to gain international acclaim and impress public opinion. However, Amalek did not seek glory, as it attacked only the weaklings, "all those who were enfeebled in your rear when you were faint and weary" (Deut. 25:18). One does not rest on his laurels if he wins a war against weak people.

Why, then, did Amalek attack the Jews? In truth, it was not a war against the ex-slaves; it was, rather, a war with the God of Israel. It attempted to destroy the people who carried the word of God. Amalek's central article of faith was: Do not fear God (see Deut. 25:18). As a matter of fact, Amalek was not motivated by fear at all. It could not tolerate the mere fact that

somebody (whether an individual or a multitude) was successful and happy. Amalek lived on envy and hate.

There are people who must love somebody; they have to pour
their love on another. To exist for them means to love, to help,
to cultivate friendship. Such a person was Abraham. Other people must hate. For them, to exist means to despise and to
destroy. These sadists will search for people upon whom they
can unleash their psychopathic hate. They wait for the innocent
victim in dark alleys and in bleak, deserted places. Amalek was
a nation of haters, of destroyers. They had heard rumors that
the Children of Israel had been freed from Egypt and immediately decided to make this people the target of their endless
hate. They got excited like a predatory beast at the sight of an
animal-victim. The tiger leaped into the herd.

How can we understand Amalek within the metaphysical
context of creation? Is Amalek the child of one who was created
in the image of God? If he is, a serious question arises: how can
one who has a divine spark enjoy the other fellow's misery and
pain; how can one center one's life around inflicting harm upon
fellow man?

The answer is given by the *Zohar* (*Bereishit* 55a). We read in
Genesis (5:1–3): "This is the book of the generations of Adam. In
the day that God created man, in the likeness of God made He
him. . . . And Adam lived a hundred years and thirty years and
begot a son in his own likeness after his image and called his
name Seth . . ." Only Seth was endowed with the likeness of
Adam, which reflected the image of God. Prior to the birth of
Seth, Adam begot children who did not bear the image of God.
These children were *toledot de-tohu*, the generation of *tohu*, of
formlessness and chaos. In other words, not all of humanity was
necessarily created in the image of God. Adam and Eve were
formed in His image. However, the image was not a grant or
ready-made charisma which was implanted in them. The image
is rather a challenge to which man is supposed to respond, a destination toward which one may journey, an ideal to be realized.

Humans are free to reject the gift of the *imago Dei,* of having been created in God's image, since acknowledging the gift imposes a heavy burden on them. However, when one declines to accept this responsibility, one does not remain a neutral being, neither divine nor evil. There is no neutrality or in-between position in the world. One belongs either to the order of creation—the order of form and constructiveness which God declares to be very good—or to the realm of *tohu va-vohu,* darkness and an abyss, of nonbeing. One is free to act either as a child of creation in the image of God or as a child of *tohu* given to destruction and the promotion of sorrow and suffering. Amalek chose the second alternative.

In biblical times, the name Amalek referred to a racial entity, to some nomadic tribe. However, the Amalek whom the Almighty swore to destroy is not a transient entity but an intrinsically stable, endless streak in creation. Only at the end of times will the Almighty defeat Amalek. The disposal of Amalek is bound up with the redemption of creation; its complete destruction will occur at the eschatological end, when the world will be purged and cleansed of evil and pain. Redemption equals the filling in of gaps in creation which the Almighty left to man, to his initiative and creativity.

The *toledot de-tohu,* the generations of chaos, are out to destroy creation *in toto.* They hate creation and want the world to return to its aboriginal state of chaos and darkness. Knowingly or unknowingly, they cannot tolerate the beauty, regularity, and orderliness which the act of creation has imposed upon formless matter. They hate the law, moral or natural, which stands in the way.

At times, the *toledot de-tohu* are successful; for a while they replace the orderliness and goodness in creation. According to the kabbalists, disease, death, famine, earthquake, or any other natural disaster—including events which are easily explained in scientific terms—are the result of a temporary takeover by the *toledot de-tohu,* who cause evil, destruction, and havoc.

Jewish history is well acquainted with individuals who, instead of representing the divine image, become the messengers of chaos. The Jews of the Persian Empire had an encounter with such a one. They fortunately succeeded in defeating him. Our generation was not so fortunate. We lost six million Jews during the several years of the reign of terror by the *toledot de-tohu*.

If Amalek represented humanity, it would mean that the Torah is good only for a small number of people. The great vision of a redeemed world would never become a reality. Therefore it was necessary to introduce a different representative of humanity, a non-Jew, Jethro, the priest of Midian. Jethro was the opposite of Amalek. If it was possible for there to be one Jethro, it is also possible for there to be others like him. Thus the great vision need not vanish because of the destructive impact of Amalek.

Jethro was the first person to praise the name of God in connection with the Exodus. The Gemara says, "It was shameful for Moses and Aaron and the six hundred thousand Jews that they did not bless [the Almighty] until Jethro came and did so" (*Sanhedrin* 94a). Of course, they said *shirah* after the miracle at the Red Sea, but not at the Exodus. There is not a single reference to the Exodus in the Song at the Sea. But Jethro came and said, "Blessed be the Lord, who has delivered you out of the hand of Egypt, and out of the hand of Pharaoh, who has delivered the people from under the hand of Egypt" (Ex. 18:10).

Not only was Jethro the first who reacted with a hymn of praise to the great event of Exodus. He intuitively anticipated the hierarchical judicial system which the Torah later recommended. Indeed, the Torah portrays Jethro in positive terms to such an extent that Moses did not want to part with him. He begged Jethro to stay to be the guiding spirit, to be our eyes, to foresee things that we would not (Num. 10:31).

Interesting is the fact that the Gemara (*Bava Metzia* 30b) derives the laws of *hesed* and *tzedakah* from a statement by Jethro: "And you shall teach them the ordinances and the *torot*, and shall show them the way in which they must walk and the actions that they must do" (Ex. 18:20). The last phrase refers to *lifnim mi-shurat ha-din,* going beyond the letter of the law. The whole concept of *hesed*, the beautiful vision of Judaism, was formulated by Jethro!

The Jewish people are a *mamlekhet kohanim*, a community of priests who teach by practicing the morality and ethics of Judaism. If our ethical deeds are good, they inspire others and bring them closer to us. But the first experience of the Jews with Amalek was a very discouraging one. It simply destroyed our vision of having the Torah become the great book of mankind, because if mankind is represented by Amalek, then mankind will never be ready for conversion.

However, there are people like Jethro, who can be taught. That is why the story of Jethro was placed in the Torah just before the story of *mattan Torah*. Because there was a man like Jethro, the whole character of *mattan Torah* assumed cosmic proportions and universal significance. Jethro could convince Moses that the world did not consist exclusively of Amalek. There are indeed people who will be ready when the proper time comes, when the hour strikes. At that time, mankind will be ready to practice the Torah and to recognize God as "King over the whole earth."

❧ Justice, Peace, and Charity: Moses as Judge

I t came to pass on the morrow (*mi-moharat*) that Moses sat to judge the people (*lishpot et ha-am*), and they stood around him from morning till evening. And when Moses' father-in-law [Jethro] saw all that Moses was doing for the people, he said, "What is this you are doing for the people? Why do you sit alone [as judge] while all the people stand around you from morning till evening?" (Ex. 18:13–14).

Jethro criticized Moses because he did not understand Moses' role as a judge—indeed, the role of any judge in Jewish jurisprudence. In the Judaic table of ethical virtues, *mishpat*, justice, occupies a central position. It is a divine attribute which is at the same time an ethical objective to be attained by man. Judaism has a unique approach to *mishpat*, and to understand it, let us first analyze the textual clue given us in the word *mi-moharat*, which opens this passage.

Mi-moharat, *On the Morrow*

The term *mi-moharat* is not just a time designation; the term contains an axiological element, a value judgment. It attempts either to explain the significance of today by attaching it to yesterday, or, vice versa, to denounce yesterday by emphasizing the contrast between it and today. Let us examine three passages in which the term occurs.

> And it came to pass on the morrow, *mi-moharat*, that Moses said unto the people: "You have sinned a great sin" . . . and when the people heard the evil tidings, they mourned (Ex. 32:30, 33:4).

In this context *mi-moharat* is used for the purpose of contrasting the today with the yesterday. Yesterday the people went berserk; today the people sobered up. Yesterday was the day of addiction to vulgar carnal pleasure, of orgiastic merrymaking, of abominable pagan rites; today is the day of awakening, of reckoning, of regaining the moral perspective. Yesterday was a day of forgetfulness and obsession; today is a day of recollection and enlightenment, and, hence, a day of mourning, of repentance, shame, and contrition. In short, *mi-moharat* signifies discontinuity, disruption of the time continuum, differentiation of human time awareness, the incommensurateness of the today with the yesterday, the miraculous metamorphosis from a sinful to a penitent community.

The phrase which the Torah employs in the chapter dealing with the spies in order to portray the change which came over the people in the course of one night is not *mi-moharat* but "*va-yashkimu va-boker*, and they rose up early in the morning," which is semantically the equivalent of *mi-moharat*.

> And they rose up early in the morning and went up to the top of the mountain, saying: "Lo, we are here and will

go up to the place which the Lord has promised, for we have sinned" (Num. 14:40).

The night before was one of mortal fear and black despair; last night they felt trapped, with all avenues of escape sealed off: "And the people wept that night" (Num. 14:1). With the rising of the morning star, they freed themselves from the monstrous dread and suicidal resignation which had exerted an irresistible spell upon them in the impenetrable darkness of a dreary, weird night. The sun became bright and shiny, a new spiritual light went on, and many things they had not understood the night before became clear in the morning. Despair and resignation changed into faith in God and in His promises. "They rose up early in the morning" is again the story of time discontinuation, of contrasts, of the incommensurateness of time experiences, of the miraculous transformation of a nightmare into a clear day vision, the change of a cowardly mob into an enlightened people.

In both cases, the day or the night before is denounced and rejected. The *mi-moharat* contains an indictment of yesterday.

At times *mi-moharat* denotes just the opposite—changeless continuity, persistent identity of time and events, the lingering on of the experience. Then *mi-moharat* ascertains the fact that an experience quite often is not extinguished with the passage of time or with the vanishing of the day.

> And you shall count *mi-moharat* the Sabbath, from the day that you brought the sheaf of the wave offering; seven weeks shall there be complete; until *mi-moharat* the seventh week shall you count fifty days (Lev. 23:15–16).

The day following the festival is not an ordinary day. The day is not just another bleak, dreary, undistinguished day. No, the day is "the morrow of the Sabbath," a continuation of the holiday. It is endowed with charisma, a specific meaning; it radiates an iridescent light; it reflects the glory of yesterday, the beauty of the Sabbath, since today and yesterday are identical.

Here, the importance of today lies in its attachment to yesterday. In this context, the biblical *mi-mohorat* is always related to a day following a holiday, to an ordinary day which is next to the holy day. By using the term *mi-moharat* we manifest our clinging to sanctity and our refusal to part with it. We arrest and keep the sanctity prisoner: "*Isru hag ba-avotim*, bind the festival with heavy ropes" (Ps. 118:27)—do not let the festival go! We call the next day *Isru Hag*. The festival is a captive!

Many halakhic institutions express the idea of the *mi-moharat* of ceaseless continuity. The most prominent is the one pertaining to *tosefet Shabbat*, adjoining time to the Sabbath. A Jew extends the Sabbath. He rushes into the Sabbath with impatience, but he is very slow to part with her. The next day is not just a day but *mi-moharat ha-Shabbat*; it is, if not endowed with intrinsic sanctity, at least appended to sanctity.

In light of the above, we understand our rabbis' comments on *mi-moharat* in our text. Rashi and Nahmanides cite the *Mekhilta* (*Masekhta de-Amalek*, chap. 1), which explains that it was *mi-moharat Yom ha-Kippurim*, the day after Yom Kippur. In other words, the phrase *mi-moharat* is not to be understood as related to the event which the Torah recorded in the preceding chapter, the arrival of Jethro, but to another event, namely, the arrival of Moses after having spent one hundred and twenty days on the top of Sinai, on the morrow of Yom Kippur.

The Jew does not just observe Yom Kippur; he experiences it as the great day of reconciliation on which God and man meet, the day of God-man companionship. "Before the Lord shall you be purified" (Lev. 16:30). But the glorious experience does not disappear immediately with the conclusion of the fast. It lives on and accompanies man into the profane, practical, and cynical world. The idea of Yom Kippur has a cathartic influence on man's awareness, enriches his personality, and sensitizes his heart. The experience of Yom Kippur and its philosophy are not abandoned with the sunset on that day. The experience lingers on and keeps company with the Jew as a living *mi-moharat* throughout the entire year.

"It came to pass on the morrow, *mi-moharat*, that Moses sat to judge the people." It was on the morrow of Yom Kippur. Why was it necessary for the Torah to single out the *mohorat* as the day of judgment? Apparently, Yom Kippur and justice are inter-related or interdependent. A judge must not mete out justice on an ordinary day. There is, in the Jewish calendar, only one day which is fit for judging people and for the rendering of just verdicts, namely, *mi-moharat Yom ha-Kippurim*. In order to understand the interrelatedness of justice and Yom Kippur we must inquire into the nature of justice as the Halakhah understands it.

Halakhic Justice

There is a strange and enigmatic institution within the halakhic civil law system, an institution unknown to the so-called *justitia civilis*, be it Roman law or English common law. I do not know of any system of law which concurs with the Halakhah concerning this enigmatic institution. I have in mind the institution of *bitzua* or *pesharah*—the notion of compromise. A profound analysis of the whole institution of *pesharah*, both at a juridic as well as at an ethico-metaphysical level, will cast a new light upon the very essence of justice the way Judaism understands it. The institution has been attacked by Jewish *maskilim* ("enlightened" thinkers). We all know the story by Sholem Aleichem about the naive rabbi of Kasrilevka who always, in any litigation, recommends a *pesharah*, half for one party and half for the other. Sholem Aleichem ridiculed the institution of *pesharah* because of ignorance and insensitivity.

What is the difference between the halakhic institution of *pesharah* and arbitration in civil law? According to the philosophy of the *justitia civilis*, a justice is appointed to render legal decisions, to resolve every controversy by informing the concerned parties who is right and who is wrong. The information is based on the judge's study and understanding of the law. The very moment he recommends a compromise, he liquidates his own role as judge and terminates the judicial process. The controversy is then settled out of court. There is no rule enjoining the justice to recommend arbitration. The judge's job is to speak on behalf of an abstract, objective, and completely uninvolved law and not to suggest other means of settling a dispute.

According to our viewpoint, *pesharah* or *bitzua* is not to be found outside but within the law. " 'Justice, justice shall you pursue' (Deut. 16:20)—one [mention of justice] refers to *din*, one to *pesharah*" (*Sanhedrin* 32b). The *dayyan*, rabbinic judge, is charged with the task of not only rendering strict legal decisions but also of settling any dispute by arbitration. The latter is a Torah solution, like the strict legal verdict. Once the parties submit to arbitration, the matter is handled by the *dayyan* in his capacity as judge. *Bitzua* or *pesharah* is not just a convenient way to end a long and difficult litigation but the ideal legal solution of any dispute. It is the religious duty of the *dayyan* to direct the judicial process toward *pesharah*. Otherwise he is derelict in discharging his duties.

We accept the view that *pesharah* requires a *kinyan*, a formal act of acquisition (*Sanhedrin* 6a; Rambam, *Hilkhot Sanhedrin* 22:6; *Shulhan Arukh*, *Hoshen Mishpat* 12:7). The *kinyan* sets up the court as the legal authority, but there is no direct obligation on the part of the litigants to give up or to renounce certain amounts of money. The Tosafot (*Sanhedrin* 6a, s.v. *tzerikhah*) already noticed that in a case of direct assumption of indebtedness, the plaintiff would require no formal acquisition, since he is in a position to exercise *mehilah*, to forgo the money, which is not subject to an acquisition. On the other hand, as far as the defendant is concerned, formal acquisition would not suffice, since it is a commitment to an indeterminate value, a *davar she-eino katzuv*, which falls under the category of

asmakhta, a transaction lacking proper intent due to unantici-
pated loss.

The *pesharah* is not a product of negotiation between the
parties, but of judicial action, of the application of a strict legal
procedure consisting of hearing and sifting evidence, listening
to arguments, ascertaining the facts, and formulating the exact
viewpoint of the law. It is a judicial act identical with any *pesak
din* (judicial ruling). The litigants, after having agreed to accept
the compromise, have no share in the making of the judgment.
Everything is determined by the judges, and all procedural
technical details are applicable to *pesharah* and *din* alike. In a
word, *pesharah* and *din* are two aspects of judicial action. The
only difference is that in the case of *din Torah* the *dayyan* consults the *Hoshen Mishpat*, while in case of *pesharah* he consults
the latter and his conscience as well.

The philosophy which underlies the institution of *pesharah*
is a twofold one. One component is ethical-metaphysical, while
the other is of an ethical-social nature. The Talmud (*Sanhedrin*
6b) derives the whole idea of *bitzua* or *pesharah* from two verses: the verse in II Samuel (8:15): "David practiced justice and
charity toward all his people," and the verse in Zechariah (8:16):
"Execute truth and the judgment of peace in your gates."

> R. Joshua ben Korhah says: It is a mitzvah to practice
> *bitzua*, for it is written, "Execute truth and the judgment
> of peace (*mishpat shalom*) in your gates." Surely where
> there is strict justice (*mishpat*) there is no peace
> (*shalom*), and where there is peace there is no strict jus-
> tice! But what is the kind of justice with which peace
> abides? We must say: *bitzua*. So it was in the case of
> David, as we read, "And David practiced justice and
> charity (*mishpat u-tzedakah*) toward all his people."
> Surely where there is strict justice (*mishpat*) there is no
> charity (*tzedakah*), and where there is charity, there is

no justice! But what is the kind of justice with which abides charity? We must say: *bitzua*.

In other words, there is a great dichotomy within the table of moral virtues, namely, the dichotomy of justice and peace, and there is also another dichotomy, of justice and charity. Both contradictions are reconciled in *bitzua*. The latter is the synthesis of justice and peace on the one hand, and of justice and charity on the other hand. Judaism knows of charitable justice or justice in charity. In contradistinction to the *justitia civilis*, Judaism proclaims *mishpat shalom*, the justice of peace.

In short, there is a double goal which *pesharah* pursues: first, justice-charity, and second, justice-peace. Let us first examine justice-charity. In the halls of *justitia civilis*, one of the parties involved in litigation gets hurt, at times badly hurt. Matters of litigation are resolved with victory for one and humiliating defeat for the other. *Justitia civilis* accepts the Aristotelian principle of contradiction in the same fashion as did classical physics. Hence *justitia civilis* knows that in every case of litigation one of the litigants is right while the other is wrong. The party that is right wins; the party that is wrong loses. Both victory and loss are total.

Judaism, which has never accepted the Aristotelian principle of contradiction, and whose Halakhah quite often recognizes both the thesis and the antithesis as true, looks upon civil conflict from a different viewpoint. A human being cannot be completely right. He is finite, a bounded being. Finitude and limitedness spell imperfection not only in the intellectual but also in the ethico-moral realm. The conclusion from this theological premise is obvious. Since the human being cannot be unqualifiedly right, his opponent or adversary cannot be absolutely wrong. They are both wrong or both right. I would prefer the first inference: two human beings involved in litigation or a civil suit are both wrong. The words of the Torah, "They shall justify the righteous, and condemn the wicked" (Deut. 25:1), should be interpreted in relative, not absolute, terms.

Therefore, Judaism tries to protect both litigants against the disgrace and humiliation of total guilt and defeat. Judaism hates malicious joy and refuses to let one of the litigants enjoy total victory and rejoicing, not so much in his winning the case as in the fact that his opponent is humiliated. Justice-charity, *mishpat u-tzedakah*, requires that the resolving of a controversy must not result in complete victory or full defeat. At the level of justice-charity there is no victor, nor is there a vanquished party. Both win; both lose. Both give something away. Both are defeated; or, if you wish to substitute another phrase, I would say both win. The judge is concerned with both and does not let the juridically right party defeat the juridically wrong party.

The Bible always associates the administration of justice with the altar: "If a man sin against his neighbor . . . and he come and swear before Your altar in this house, then hear You in heaven, and do, and judge Your servants" (I Kings 8:31–32). The section of *Parashat Mishpatim* (Ex. 21 ff.) dealing with the administration of justice is a continuation of the previous section in *Yitro* (Ex. 20:21–23) concerned with the construction of the altar. Why? In order to teach you that the judges must sit near the altar (Rashi, Ex. 21:1, drawing on the *Mekhilta*). There is no justice without sacrifice.

Mishpat Shalom, *The Judgment of Peace*

Bitzua is also nurtured by the idea of *mishpat shalom*. *Justitia civilis* is concerned with resolving a conflict but not with reconciliation of the people involved in the conflict. That is not the job of the judge. Hatred deepens and antagonism increases in the courtrooms and halls of civil justice. Feelings of enmity and vindictiveness may intensify, yet justice does not care about its failure to restore friendships or to bring people closer to each other. *Shalom*, peace, is outside the halls of justice; it is up to the social worker, if he or she can do the job.

Judaism, by urging both parties to abate their claims and to retreat from their points of vantage, has changed the role of a *dayyan* from a magistrate into that of a teacher who tells both parties that their respective claims are absurd. The judge makes the litigants understand that neither of them is totally right or totally wrong. It dawns upon both parties that hostility and hate are out of place, and that the whole conflict was not worth the emotional excitement it generated. As a result of the *dayyan*'s intervention, peace and friendship are re-established. Again, it is justice before the altar, because the altar is not only the symbol of sacrifice but also the symbol of peace and reconciliation: One may not raise his sword upon the altar (Ex. 20:22). Justice before the altar means both justice in charity and justice in peace.

This philosophy comes to expression in the famous saying in *Avot* (1:8):

> Yehudah ben Tabbai says: [When serving as a judge] do not act as *orekhei ha-dayyanim*; when the litigants stand before you, consider them both as guilty; but when they are dismissed from you, consider them both as innocent, provided they have accepted the judgment.

In modern Hebrew, *orekh din* means an attorney. But Yehudah ben Tabbai is not saying that a judge may not advocate for one party against the other. That would be plain corruption, *ivvut ha-din*. Instead, I would translate his admonition as: Do not act like an omniscient judge who renders his decisions with a feeling of absolute certitude. The term *orekh din* is an attribute of the Almighty. The prayer recited on Rosh Ha-Shanah and Yom Kippur, *le-E-l orekh din*, refers to God, to whom justice is as clear as is a set table, a *shulhan arukh*, to those who want to enjoy the food before them.

Orekh din means an all-knowing judge. Yehudah ben Tabbai once thought of himself in such terms, and he committed murder on account of it. He sentenced to death an *ed zomem*, a type of false witness, who did not deserve to be executed (*Hagigah* 16b, *Makkot* 5b). He speaks from experience: Only the Almighty is an all-knowing judge. A human must not approach a case with the sense of absolute knowledge and absolute certainty. Humility on the part of the judge is the first prerequisite. He cannot determine guilt and innocence. The philosophy of *pesharah* recommends a paradoxical approach. First, tell the litigants that they are both wrong and hence that both must make amends and abate something of their claims. After they have agreed to give up, pronounce both of them right. This is justice before the altar. Is not this doctrine nurtured by the sublime idea of confession and atonement on Yom Kippur?

Moses judged only *mi-mohorat Yom ha-Kippurim*. He always remembered, while he was sitting in judgment, that to practice *mishpat* and act like a *shofet*, one must be aware of the Yom Kippur outlook on guilt and innocence, on crime, punishment, and reconciliation. The day of judgment must always fall on the morrow of Yom Kippur, appended to the day that symbolizes par excellence the ideals of the judicial action: grace and love. On Yom Kippur, a sinner burdened with crime and injustice comes before God, who purges him. A person is never completely wicked and corrupt. There is something good in him. It might be hidden in the inner recesses of his personality, it might be concealed even from himself; but there is something good in him, and therefore the Holy One opens the gates of repentance to him. That is how a judge should look upon the people who appear before him. Any day on which Moses played the role of a justice was *mi-mohorat*, attached to Yom Kippur or to the experience he lived through on Mount Sinai when the Almighty descended in a pillar of cloud.

The Meaning of Shafot

At this juncture we arrive at a very important conclusion. We see that the term *shafot* does not denote judicial activity exclusively. The semantics of *shafot* are all-inclusive and point toward the totality of human relations. *Shafot* means to have concern, to advise, to be preoccupied with certain needs, to help, to save, to fight, and to be together.

That *shafot* represents more than mere judging, and that it embraces the whole gamut of human relations, becomes obvious when we read the psalms of *Kabbalat Shabbat*. For instance,

> The heavens will be glad and the earth will rejoice, the sea and its fullness will roar; the field and everything in it will exult, then all the trees of the forest will sing with joy—before God, for He will have arrived, He will have arrived *lishpot ha-aretz*, to judge the earth. He will judge the earth with righteousness, and peoples with His truth (Ps. 96:11–13).

If the Almighty is coming to judge the world, then fear and awe (as described in *U-netanneh tokef*), not joy, song, and ecstatic gladness, are in place. Similarly,

> Zion will hear and be glad, and the daughters of Judah will exult, because of Your judgments, Lord (Ps. 97:8).

> The sea and its fullness will roar, the world and those who dwell therein. Rivers will clap hands, mountains will exult together—before God, for He will have arrived to judge the earth (Ps. 98:7–9).

When God judges creation, who can say that he will not be found wanting? "Should You mete out the full measure of justice, who would be cleared before You?" (*Mussaf*, first day of Rosh Ha-Shanah).

The answer to these questions is to be found in the multiple semantics of the verb *shafot*. "For He has come *lishpot* the earth" means that God is coming to commune with this world;

He will come close to creation from the transcendental distances, from the mysterious beyond, to establish contact, show concern and interest, involve Himself in the destiny of man in general and of His elect community in particular. The nearness of the Creator to His creation, the closeness of man to God, inspires endless joy and rapture. What is more exalted and what is more sublime than to feel the touch of Infinity on one's shoulder? Clearly, *shafot* does not have here the sense of judging.

In Greek, Latin, and English translation, the name of the book *Shofetim* is rendered as the Book of Judges. This translation is erroneous; it should be the Book of Leaders. We are told: "Now Deborah the prophetess, the wife of Lapidot, she *shofetah* Israel at that time . . . and the children of Israel came up to her for *mishpat*" (Judg. 4:4–5). If all Deborah had to do was resolve civil conflicts and render judicial decisions, then why did she act like a ruling queen? Nothing is told about her supposedly main preoccupation of judging. We read instead of Deborah's dedication to the people and her political authority. She declared war on Sisera; she chose the commander-in-chief who led the Israelite troops against the legions of Sisera; she personally accompanied Barak to the field of battle; she sang the great hymn of joy and praise.

Does a magistrate do all these things? Certainly not! She was more than a justice; she was a queen, leader, teacher, and friend of the people. Indeed, she says what she was: "Until I arose, a mother in Israel" (Judg. 5:7). In light of this we should translate *hi shofetah* (4:4) not as "she judged," but as "she led, guided, and taught the children of Israel at that time." She was their mother. Similarly, "and the children of Israel came up to her for *mishpat*" (4:5) means that they came up to her for guidance, counsel, and advice. The same is true of all the "judges"; they not only judged but taught and guided. "And Samuel *shafat* Israel all the days of his life" (I Sam. 7:15)—Samuel guided the destiny of Israel all his life. So it was with Moses.

Moses as Judge

Let us now ask a simple question. Why were there so many litigants that Moses had to stand the whole day sitting in judgment? The Jews in the desert were provided with food, clothes, and all other necessities; there was no need for them to win their daily bread by the sweat of their brows. "He fed you the manna. . . . Your raiment grew not old upon you, nor did your foot swell" (Deut. 8:4). There was no commerce, no manufacturing of goods, no competition. There was no place for commercial feuds, for economic conflicts. If somebody tried to hoard the manna, he was punished at once. The manna bred worms and rotted. If one attempted to grab more than the ratio allotted to him, by the time he came home from picking the manna, the additional measure disappeared. In short, cheating, grabbing, and stealing were impossibilities. The whole sentence, "And Moses sat *lishpot* the people . . . from morning till evening," is mystifying.

However, the puzzle is cleared up with a change in the semantics of *shafot*. If *shafot* denotes the total spectrum of human relations, beginning with leadership but concluding with love, concern, and unqualified friendship, then we understand what Moses did. There was not much need for judicial action because litigation was minimal. However, there was a great and awesome need for leadership, for teaching, and, particularly, for giving friendship. There were many human tragedies which confronted Moses and demanded his attention. People had been in slavery for hundreds of years, ridiculed, humiliated, tortured; their wives had been dishonored not just once, their children snatched from motherly arms and brutally murdered. Suddenly they were liberated, and many did not know how to live in freedom. Nightmares pursued them; memories played havoc with them; each knock on the door at night reminded them of the blood-chilling scenes of a few years before.

The people were completely dislocated mentally, displaced physically, confused and frightened. They needed somebody to lead and teach them, somebody in whom they could confide. They clung to Moses and wanted to be in his company. His mere presence was inspiring for them, his ways were reassuring and calming, his words of wisdom enlightening, driving away all the ghosts of the past. His words of comfort and solace placated their pent-up perplexed emotions, healed their schisms and fused them with hope and faith: "The people stood around Moses from the morning to the evening" (Ex. 18:13). They stood about him because they loved him and were fascinated by him; they could not be separated from him. The standing was not of a ceremonial nature at all; it was natural, almost instinctual.

Jethro misunderstood all this. He could not imagine a person who was capable of being a justice, teacher, and friend all at the same time. He thought that Moses played the role of a stern ruler, a mighty king in whose presence no one was allowed to sit. As Rashi (Ex. 18:13) comments, Jethro thought that the people stood because they were instructed to do so, because protocol demanded it. This was distasteful to Jethro in that he thought Moses had made light of the respect due to Israel, and he therefore reproved him for sitting while the people stood.

Of course, Jethro was wrong. Moses certainly did not make light of the respect due to Israel. Moses loved the people; he breathed and died for them. The people's standing was not commanded but spontaneous; they stood in order to be close to their great teacher and friend, to be able to touch his garment. Interestingly, the Torah uses the verb *a-m-d* to describe the scene ("The people stood [*va-ya'amod*] around Moses from morning till evening," Ex. 18:13), but Jethro uses the verb *n-tz-v* in his rebuke ("Why do you sit alone while all the people stand around you from morning till evening?" Ex. 18:14). The verb *a-m-d* simply describes a physical posture. However, the verb *n-tz-v* means to be prepared to serve: "Then Joseph could not restrain himself before all them that stood (*nitzavim*) before him" (Gen. 45:1). The Bible uses the term *nitzavim* to emphasize that those people were subservient to Joseph. Jethro accused Moses of acting like a ruler, while Moses, in fact, acted like a teacher and friend.

Moses answers Jethro and explains his threefold role: (a) "The people come to me to inquire of God"; (b) "When they have a matter they come to me, and I judge between a man and his fellow"; (c) "I make them know the statutes of God and His laws" (Ex. 18:15–16). Nahmanides explains that the first sentence refers to prayer. The people in time of distress and crisis come to me with the request that I intercede with the Almighty on their behalf. The second sentence is related to judging "between a man and his fellow." When they have a conflict or controversy, they come to me for judgment or guidance and I fulfill my task. According to the *Mekhilta*, Moses hints here at two options: " 'Between a man'—this refers to judgment without *pesharah*; 'and his fellow'—this refers to judgment with *pesharah*, for the two litigants depart as friends." The meaning of the third sentence is obvious: Moses is the great teacher who instructs the people in the divine law and doctrines.

Moses, in other words, is the friend who shares in the people's travails and joys; the leader who administers not ruthless *justitia civilis* but divine righteousness tempered with love and grace; and the educator who enlightens and trains a whole people, fathers and mothers, sons and daughters.

Rashi concurs with Nahmanides that Moses had three tasks. They differ only as to the order in which the tasks are enumerated. According to Rashi's interpretation, Moses is first of all a teacher: "The people come to me to inquire of God," to seek instruction from the Almighty. Second, Moses is a friend who helps the people in times of need: "When they have a matter," when they face adversity, "*ba elai*, he [in the singular] comes to me"—each individual is free to knock on my door at any time of the day or the night and to tell me his sad story. Third, "I judge between a man and his fellow, and I make them know the statutes of God and His laws"—Moses is a judge who settles disputes and resolves controversies, and at the same time teaches as well.

Nahmanides combines the first part of the sentence, "When they have a matter (*davar*) they come to me," with the second part, "I judge between a man and his fellow." The full verse expresses one idea—namely, judging. *Davar* in this interpretation signifies a controversy. Rashi divides the verse into two parts. "When they have a matter they come to me" refers most probably to prayer (*davar* = trouble), and "I judge between a man and his fellow" refers to judging, which is simultaneously teaching as well. While Nahmanides separates "When they have a matter . . . I judge" from the last part of "I do make them know," since the latter is concerned with pure teaching, Rashi finds teaching mentioned at the very beginning—"The people come to me to inquire of God."

In Judaism, there is a strange equation: to judge = to teach; to teach = to pray; to pray = to love. Moses engaged in all three. It is obvious that it is impossible to teach if there is no reciprocal love and commitment between teacher and student. The intellect does not respond and the student freezes up; his mind closes and the teacher finds it very hard to penetrate inside. It is also self-evident that love and sympathy are indispensable for prayer. How can one pray for someone else if one does not share in his travail and one is not involved in his suffering?

Hence the most paradoxical equation emerges: to judge = to love. Of course a modern jurist will laugh at this ancient equation. Notwithstanding the ridicule, the equation is true. Justice can only be achieved before the altar, for the latter is the place of love and sacrifice. This is what Moses tells Jethro: I am their judge, but that means to teach, to love, and to pray for them.

Judging from Morning till Evening

Is it really possible [that Moses sat in judgment the whole day long]? But the explanation is that any judge who gives a just decision as truth demands it, even though he spends but one hour on it, Scripture accounts it to him as though he had occupied himself with the study of the Torah the whole day long; and as though he became co-partner with the Almighty in the work of creation, of which it is stated (Gen. 1:5), "It was evening and it was morning, the first day" (Rashi, Ex. 18:13, s.v. *min*).

Rashi quotes the *Mekhilta*. However, in our text of the *Mekhilta* the first answer is not mentioned (nor does the Gemara in *Shabbat* 10a make mention of it). Rashi is trying to put across the thought that judging and teaching are identical acts. Moreover, the impact of instruction through handling a case properly and through delivering a true and fair verdict is far greater than the impact of theoretical teaching. An hour of true, honest judging is as productive and significant as a full day's teaching by mouth.

But what is being taught through judging: is it justice-charity or justice-peace? What do the litigants learn? What outlook on life is put across to them?

Judging teaches the idea of "*Va-yehi erev va-yehi boker*, It was evening and it was morning." Ibn Ezra as well as Nahmanides and Kimhi expounded that the term *erev*, evening, is derived from *arev*, to mix or to confuse, and that the term *boker*, morning, is derived from *baker*, to discriminate or distinguish. *Erev*, writes Ibn Ezra (Gen. 1:5, s.v. *erev*), "is close in meaning to *hoshekh*, darkness. *Erev* is so called because forms are then intermingled. The opposite of evening is called *boker* because one can then distinguish between various forms." Nahmanides (s.v. *va-yikra*) writes: "The beginning of the night is called *erev* because shapes of things appear confused in it, and the beginning of the day is called *boker* because then a man can distinguish between various forms, as explained by Rabbi Abraham [ibn Ezra]." Kimhi (Gen. 1:8, s.v. *va-yehi*) expresses himself in identical fashion:

The time of the setting of the sun is called *erev*, from the term for admixture (*hit'arvut*) and combination of matter, for it is a time of darkness, and matters are mixed, for man cannot differentiate or distinguish between things. . . . The beginning of the day is called *boker*, from the term for investigation and analysis, *bikkoret*, for in the morning everything can be analyzed by the light of the day.

There are two streams of being: that of rationality and that of mystery. Reality is both intelligible and a *mysterium magnum*, never to be unraveled. The simplicity of the mathematical equation which answers the question of how the universe functions, and the insoluble philosophical and metaphysical enigma as regards the question of what the universe is and why it is— these are characteristic of being. Nature, at times, is very cooperative, smilingly opening up to us her recesses, allowing man to climb to the stars, in motherly fashion revealing to us her secrets; at other times the same nature is tough and ruthless, refusing to recognize our presence, closed up, defying man's aspirations, letting him confront the *mysterium magnum* in fear and trembling. Being, as such, contains both *erev*, confusion, and *boker*, clarity; a mixture (*ta'arovet*) as well as distinctiveness; progress which defies the imagination and humiliating stagnation and immobility.

This dual streak in reality, with which science has to reckon, is also significant to the individual. The private human existential experience is a dual one. The human "day," the human existence in time, is not a uniform one. It is split into two parts, two dimensions, one called *boker* and the other *erev*. We live in the dimension of understanding and discriminating, where the existential awareness is a rational one and the ontological experience is saturated with joy and happiness. We exist, and it seems to us that we also comprehend the meaning of our living in time. It is a redeemed existence; we are cognizant of our continuous growth, intellectual as well as emotional, with the passage of time. What we did not know yesteryear or yesterday we know today; and what appears to us puzzling today, will be clear and simple tomorrow. We move with time toward greater goods and more enchanting horizons. Time means enlightenment, *boker* equals *bakor*. The morning is so bright and so beautiful. Man is the victor!

However, there is another part to the existential experience of man, when the existential awareness turns into existential confusion and nonunderstanding, when the ontological consciousness mocks and denies itself. Contradictions show up wherever harmony prevailed before. What was united is split. Everything seems topsy-turvy. There is no integrity. We just pick up the debris of a shattered existence. Events happen seemingly without any rationale; the whole act of living becomes a very ugly affair. You ask why and what, and you find no answer. This kind of existence, which was so beautifully defined by R. Eliezer ha-Kappar as an unwanted compulsory existence from which man paradoxically is liberated by an unwanted compulsory death, "Without your will you live, and without your will you die" (*Avot* 4:22), is the *erev* part of the human lifespan.

Judaism taught man to accept both the *erev* and the *boker* dimensions of our existential experience, to be bold in the morning and humble in the evening, to be grateful for the morning, when everything is orderly and neatly arranged, and to be faithful at the eventide, when everything is in utter confusion and disorder. Man is victor-conqueror in the morning; he is then the critic, the expert scientist. He likes this role, of course! However, he should also learn to like the reverse role, in which man is defeated by nature; in which he is not the critic, since he cannot discriminate in the darkness; in which he is no expert but rather is perplexed; in which he does not rule, since he is perhaps the weakest living being on earth. "Man was defeated" is the motto of eventide, and this cry must be heard by man. The litigants who stand before a judge are seeking victory; they desire the *boker*. The judge who renders the true decision of justice-peace or justice-charity teaches them how to give up and accept defeat and be satisfied with the *erev*.

Moses judged from morning to evening, and always "on the morrow of Yom Kippur."

The Golden Calf and the Roots of Idolatry

"This Man Moses"

Soon after the revelation at Sinai, the Jews committed the sin of the Golden Calf. We should note that *prima facie* this sin was more abominable, more horrible, than the sin of eating of the Tree of Knowledge. If we translate it into halakhic terms, the sin of the Tree of Knowledge consisted in eating forbidden foods, while the sin of the Golden Calf touched the very essence of Judaism, namely, the prohibition against idolatry. Yet, when Adam ate from the Tree of Knowledge, all future generations were struck by disaster. Adam alienated himself from his Creator and was driven out of Paradise. According to *Hazal*, God had intended for man to live forever, but the original sin brought about death and man became mortal. When the community alienated itself from the Creator by worshipping the Golden Calf, the consequences of the sin were not as tragic.

The answer is obvious. When Adam sinned, there was nobody to pray and intercede with the Almighty on his behalf; he had no Moses. He did not know the secret of prayer and the great mystery of repentance. He considered sin as absolute, with no performance capable of erasing it. He did not know that repentance is effective, that the tear of contrition and regret washes away any sin. He did not know that the courage to admit an error is cathartic and that the admission of guilt is the finest sacrifice one may offer to the Almighty.

Not only that, but he defended his sin, blaming "the woman You gave to be with me" (Gen. 3:12). Adam did not possess the fortitude to respond to God's call, "*Ayekkah*, Where are you?" He hid himself and thought that God's voice would not penetrate the thick foliage of the tree. He made a terrible mistake.

When the community sinned, Moses knew how to meet disaster; he prayed for the people. Moreover, he taught the people how to confess. The great message of *teshuvah* was revealed with the Thirteen Attributes of Mercy, which entail the promise that God accepts the sinner, provided the latter knocks on the door and calls to God. Yom Kippur memorializes the revelation of the message of *teshuvah*, which took place on his last day on Mount Sinai. On Yom Kippur, God revealed to Moses the mystery of reconciliation between man and the Almighty. The Torah also informs us of the requirements for *teshuvah*. Regret, *haratah*, is not enough; a feeling of mourning and grief must accompany *haratah*. "When the people heard these evil tidings, they mourned and no man put on his ornaments" (Ex. 33:4).

When we compare the etiology of the first sin with that of the Golden Calf, we find that the motives are almost contradictory. Adam wanted to compete, as it were, with the Almighty. His sin was a result of pride and vanity. Apparently, he was aware that he was created in the image of the Holy One; otherwise, it never would have occurred to him to try to be like God. He knew that he was endowed with a great charisma and great ability, and he felt as if compliance with the divine norm would stymie his growth and development. On the contrary, he thought that he would become greater, more prominent, more powerful and wiser if he violated the prohibition addressed to him by the Almighty.

What, though, motivated the people to make a Golden Calf? The people had left Egypt with the help of the Almighty. They themselves witnessed the miracles which took place, first in Egypt and then at the Red Sea. They experienced the presence of God: "And they believed in the Lord and in His servant Moses" (Ex. 14:31). How can we explain this rapid change from being a people which reached great heights to a primitive band of idol worshippers and idolaters?

Ibn Ezra (Ex. 32:1, s.v. *amar*) says that the people did not mean to proclaim that the calf was God, but only that it was a successor to Moses. They felt that they themselves did not have access to the Almighty. Only somebody of great charisma and ability could have access to Him. The people sinned because they were perplexed. Moses had been gone for a long time. "This man Moses, who brought us up out of the land of Egypt, we know not what has become of him" (Ex. 32:1). They made the calf in order to replace Moses, not to replace the Almighty. They did not understand that, while Moses was the greatest of all prophets and the greatest of all men, every Jew has access to God. They did not realize that the relationship which God promised to their ancestors was independent of Moses' presence. Sometimes it is a sense of one's greatness that causes sin; sometimes it is a sense of one's smallness.

Indeed, man is great *and* small—and the reality of *teshuvah* is rooted in this inner contradiction of the human personality. Man sinned because he is small. Had he been a great being exclusively, he would not have sinned. Aaron confesses, *"Asher no'alnu va-asher hatanu"* (Num. 12:11)—we were foolish, we were small, and we sinned. However, this is as far as regret for the past is concerned. But when man wants to amend his ways and start a new life, he must have faith in himself that he is capable of doing it, that he is a hero, that he has an iron will. This double awareness, this mystery of *teshuvah*—which contains a real contradiction between man great and man small— is found in David's psalms. On the one hand, "When I behold

Your heavens, the work of Your fingers, the moon and the stars which You have ordained; what is man that You are mindful of him, and the son of man that You remember him?" (Ps. 8:4–5); and on the other, "Yet You have made him a little lower than the angels" (Ps. 8:6).

Idolatry Today

This duality can help us understand the contemporary relevance of the prohibition of idolatry. We all know that Judaism hates paganism, the polytheistic universe populated by a variety of deities and semideities. How many times does the Pentateuch warn Israel against the venal sin of idol worship! We still read twice daily: "Take heed to yourselves, lest your heart be deceived and you turn aside and serve other gods and worship them" (Deut. 11:16).

Reading the Pentateuch, one may naively say that all this was pertinent thousands of years ago, when mankind moved in the orbit of polytheism, when worship of the divine was synonymous with the lewd cultic rites of paganism. However, nowadays—when civilized religion is monotheistic, and both Christianity and Islam fundamentally accept the message of monotheism carried by the Jew—the whole problem of monotheism versus polytheism has lost its significance. Who is an idol worshipper in our midst? The relentless struggle in which Moses and our prophets engaged millennia ago is, in our age, an anachronism. People either believe in one God or they do not believe at all, instead finding delight in agnosticism or atheistic doctrines. Who professes faith in a multitude of gods?

However, when we read the prophets carefully, we discern that the prophets did not foresee the defeat of paganism at an early historical stage. They were not optimistic at all about the prospects of an easy and quick victory over polytheism. Of course, they beheld a great and fascinating vision. They were captivated by the sublime goal, the awe-inspiring destiny of man, when God will reign supreme over all nations. However, all these visions, hopes, and prophecies were related to a very distant time, to a day replete with majesty and glory, remote and beyond the reach of historical occurrence, somewhere on the fringes of time at the end of days. In short, the prophets were eschatologically minded when they spoke in glowing and passionate words of the universal kingdom of God.

Indeed, we still pray to God and plead with Him to wipe out idol worship from the face of the earth. On one of the most solemn days of the year, Rosh Ha-Shanah, we recite one of the loftiest and most impressive liturgical compositions ever written: *Ve-al Ken Nekavveh Lekha*. What is the content of this beautiful prayer if not our indomitable faith that the day—which is still far off—will come on which the human race will cast away all its idols and heathendom will be utterly destroyed?

> We therefore hope in You, O Lord our God, that we may speedily behold the glory of Your might, when You will remove the abominations from the earth and the pagan gods will be utterly obliterated . . . when the children of all flesh will call upon Your name, when You will turn to Yourself all the evildoers upon earth.

We conclude with the enigmatic words: "On that day the Lord shall be one and His name one" (Zech. 14:9). The conclusion one must derive from this prayer is that heathendom still rules our civilized world. If we are dissatisfied with the many imperfections of our social and moral order, if we encounter injustice, brutality, and cruel, ruthless stupidity, if falsehood, wickedness, violence, and evil forces are still rampant and unfettered, if man is suspicious, envious, petty, and obscene—it is only due to the fact that man is still a heathen, his life pagan and his cult idolatrous. He has not yet understood and intellectually digested the doctrine of "the Lord our God, the Lord is one" (Deut. 6:4). When and if man abandons his pagan deities and commits himself to the principle of the unity of God, he and the world will be redeemed. All Judaism wants, desires, prays, and hopes for is universal acceptance of "the Lord shall be one and His name one."

And yet, as I walk out of the synagogue on Rosh Hashanah, I have never noticed a figure of the abominable and cynical Baal with the horns, nor a statue of aging Zeus with his determined and energetic face, nor a sculpture of young Apollo with his muscular body, nor a figure of Aphrodite emerging from the foam of the onrushing tide. On the contrary, I see inscriptions on many portals referring to God the Almighty. Statesmen in their addresses mention God and invoke His blessings. The God whose grace they beg is the God of Israel, whom the Western nations have accepted. No one turns to the Baal or to Dionysius, and yet we pray that, in spite of the might of heathendom that rules humanity at present, the dawn of a new day will finally come. We assert that we are still enveloped by a dark, grisly night of pagan terror and superstition.

Judaism apparently has a different concept of paganism than the one to which the reader of history is accustomed. Paganism is not only a historical phenomenon that expressed itself in a definitive ritual, in an organized religious society, in clerical institutions and cultic forms, but also—and perhaps mainly—in a way of thinking about, feeling, and valuing things and events. Paganism is a method of measuring and assessing the worth of our experiences. It is more an axiology than a theology; it manifests itself more conspicuously in value judgments than in logical propositions, in appreciating rather than understanding.

Let me be more specific. The controversy between heathendom and Judaism revolves about one question: Who is man? Judaism, as we have seen, has developed a dialectical philosophy of man. It states, paradoxically and strangely, that man is both divine and demonic, great and small, powerful and weak, kind and cruel. Man can rise to heaven and fall into a bottom-less abyss. As we recite on the Day of Atonement:

> What are we? What are our lives? What is our piety? What is our righteousness? What our helpfulness? What our strength? What our might? What shall we say before You? Are not all the mighty men as naught before You, the men of renown as though they had not been, the wise as if without knowledge and the understanding as if without discernment? For most of their works are void, and the days of their lives are vanity before You, and the preeminence of man over the beast is naught, for all is vanity.

> Nevertheless, from the beginning You have set man apart and made him worthy of standing before You!

Our dialectical theory of man is strange, bordering on the antithetic and antinomic. Man is a dichotomous being, and both contradictory aspects are true. Using this antinomy in man as a point of departure, Judaism has developed an axiology or prac-tical philosophy. Since God has chosen man to stand before Him and surrounded him with glory and honor—in other words, since He has bestowed upon man so many gifts: intellectual capacity, mechanical skillfulness, technological aptitude, the ability to plan, to anticipate future happenings, creativity in many fields, a vivid fantasy and a powerful will—man must not waste these talents and faculties, and must utilize them to the utmost.

Hence, Judaism insists that man develop his potentialities to the fullest. The Torah encourages man to think, to work, to learn, to improve and perfect himself and his environment, and to intervene whenever necessary in natural processes, if such interference will contribute to the self-realization of man. God purposely did not complete the world; He left uneven surface lines in creation in order to offer man an opportunity to join Him in His creative gesture and become a co-participant in the mysterious act of continuous creation. Not even Jewish mysticism has preached the strange doctrine of self-effacement or the folly of quest. We have never tried to shut out of our souls all natural forms and images, and to purge the body of all carnal drives and urges. We demand of man complete involvement in all worldly affairs. We equate withdrawal from the world and society with cowardice and warn against it. Our philosophy preaches activism, aggressiveness, and articulateness. The voice of the Creator, which echoed through the spaces of a newly created world when He addressed Himself to man on that numinous sixth day of creation—"Be fruitful and multiply, and replenish the earth and subdue it" (Gen. 1:28)—is still ringing in our ears.

However, man is also small, petty, and untrustworthy; he is not only divine but satanic. Hence, he must never overreach himself. He must not admire and adore himself; he must not be too impressed with his own stature in creation. An exaggerated self-appraisal or an inflated self-awareness would lead to self-glorification, the latter being equal to self-idolization and heathenism.

"You Shall Have No Other Gods Before Me"

Who, then, is the perennial idol that man worships, the deity whom man adores, the god to whom man is unqualifiedly committed? It is man himself! The most horrible, repulsive, and menacing idolatrous worship is the deification and absolutization of man. Man may be great; but if we forget even for a fraction of a second that he is also very small, we commit the sin of idolatry. Man is divine, yet when he is not always aware of his satanic nature, he errs and is guilty of a grave offense. Absolutization of man's worth, hypostatization of his capabilities and accomplishments, idealization of his nature—these are tantamount to the most barbarous form of idolatry. The world will be rehabilitated and redeemed only when man has adopted with regard to himself a dual value judgment and looks at himself not only with admiration but with suspicion as well.

Paganism preached naivete, Judaism a critical and often skeptical approach to man and his attainments. Judaism relativizes all human finite values and aptitudes, denying them unconditional commitment. Judaism maintains that creation as such has no ontic autonomy. God is not only the creator and governor of the world in a physico-dynamic sense, whose will determines the mathematical regularity of the cosmic process in all its phases, but also the master of everything on a juridic plane. God owns His creations, the endless stretches of the universe from our small earth to the outer fringes of the cosmos. "The earth is the Lord's and the fullness thereof, the world and they that dwell therein" (Ps. 24:1). The status of man is that of tenant, a sharecropper: "For the land is Mine; for you are strangers and sojourners with Me" (Lev. 25:23).

This is the idea of the Sabbath. The Torah demands temporary withdrawal from one's daily routine so that we can shake off the hypnotic influence which material possessions exert over us and face the truth that we are managing someone's estate, not our own. In Hebrew, *Shabbat* means discontinuation, withdrawal—man retreats from something which never belonged to him, from a delusion and a mirage that the world is his.

The same is true of *tzedakah*. In all civilized countries, the state collects debts and taxes but not charity, because the very meaning of charity relates to kindness, benevolence, free giving, generosity—something which can never be enforced or imposed. However, Judaism has adopted the strange attitude that society has a right to assess a person's assets, fix the amount he is able to give away to charity, and collect it. In our historical annals we know of many cases in which rabbinical courts issued bills of foreclosure on estates because of default on the part of certain individuals to contribute generously to the charitable institutions of the respective community. The Halakhah does not distinguish between legal and charitable indebtedness. Why? Because the money one possesses is not one's own. We owe whatever we have to the Almighty— "Mine is the silver and Mine is the gold" (Hag. 2:8)—and therefore we must carry out the mandate given us by the Master.

The idea of divine ownership and mastery is not confined to material goods; it is comprehensive and universal, reaching down to the most hidden recesses of human existence. Who does not consider children his exclusive, most cherished, and most precious possession? Yet Judaism holds the view that only through the bestowal of endless divine grace can we explain the miracle of fatherhood and motherhood. No one may take this gift from heaven as something natural and ordinary. We read in the Pentateuch that Sarah, Rebecca, Rachel, and Hannah were barren for a long time. Only long prayers to God and His infinite mercy blessed them with a child. Why did God arrange matters in such a perplexing way? Why all the tribulations, suffering, and misery of these lonely women? God wanted to demonstrate that bearing children is a great divine gift and must not be taken for granted. The child does not belong to the parent; he is just entrusted to their care. He is the son of God. Hannah understood this message and called her baby Samuel, "because I have asked him (*she'iltiv*) of the Lord" (I Sam. 1:20). The verb *she'iltiv* has a twofold connotation: to ask and to borrow. We may depart from the standard translation and interpret her words as meaning, "because I have borrowed him from God."

Man does not belong to himself. All my aptitudes, capacities, talents, and capabilities are not mine; they were graciously given to me. If man understands this philosophy, then he may become truly great and stand before the Lord. If he tries to usurp power, to embezzle material goods and spiritual riches from God, then he forfeits his greatness, shrinks in personal stature, and becomes a mocking, destructive mephisto-idol.

There are many injunctions in the Bible against idol worship. But there is no injunction against atheism, because there is, in truth, no atheism. There are only two choices—the true God or an idol. When a man revolts against God, he thinks he is being flexible and free, but soon he builds himself his own idol and worships himself. On the verse "You shall have no other gods before Me" (Ex. 20:2), Rashi (s.v. *al*) comments: " 'Before Me'—that is, as long as I exist; so that you should not say that only that generation [that left Egypt] was enjoined against idolatry." This is a commandment for all generations.

"If Your Presence Go Not with Us"

The sin of the Golden Calf had an interesting impact. Earlier, Moses had not protested when God said:

> Behold, I send an angel before you to keep you in the way and to bring you to the place which I have promised you. . . . If you shall indeed obey his voice, and do all that I speak: then I will be an enemy to your enemies, and an adversary to your adversaries. For My angel shall go before you, and bring you in to the [land of the] Amorite and Hittite . . . (Ex. 23:20–23).

After the sin, God says, "Therefore, now go and lead your people to the place of which I have spoken to you, and My angel will march in front of you" (Ex. 32:34). Here, however, Moses protests:

> You said to me, Bring up this people: and You have not let me know whom You will send with me. Yet You have said, I know you by name, and you have also found favor in My sight. Now therefore I pray to You, if I have found favor in Your sight, show me now Your way, that I may know You . . . and consider that this nation is Your people.

> And He said, My presence shall go with you, and I shall give you rest.

> And he said to Him, If Your presence go not with me, carry us not up from here (Ex. 33:12–15).

Moses initially accepted God's sending an angel beforehand. Now he demands God's presence itself.

We understand all this when we realize that prior to the episode of the Golden Calf the people of Israel were not stained by sin. (The murmuring for water was a complaint and not a major sin.) Moses thought that Jewish history would never be stained with sin. In that case, there would be no need for God's *hesed*. The lodestar of the Jewish people would be truth and justice; in such a situation an angel is sufficient. An angel represents truth, *middat ha-emet*, but angels know nothing about kindness, *hesed*. It is only the Holy One Himself who combines them as *rav hesed ve-emet*. When sin became an historical reality, the presence of God Himself became indispensable. An angel does not tolerate a sin:

> Behold, I send an angel before you. . . . Take heed of him and obey his voice, provoke him not; for he will not pardon your transgressions, for My name is in him (Ex. 23:20–21).

The name that is in him, explains Rashi (23:21, s.v. *ki*), is *Sha-dai*, which represents the natural law, the mathematical equation which rules in the universe. There is no *hesed* within a universe governed by natural law. If two stars collide, both will be destroyed. The angel who represents *Sha-dai* cannot understand *middat ha-hesed* and *middat ha-teshuvah*.

Before the great sin, Moses thought that there would be no need for the presence of the Holy One Himself. But afterwards,

Moses realized that while Jewish history would be great and full of heroic deeds, it would also be a tragic history full of sin. Only God can forgive. His actual presence became a necessity.

❧ Sanctity and Sovereignty: Moses as King

"Moses Did Not Know That the Skin of His Face Shone"

In many places, the Midrash applies to Moses the verse "When there was a king in Jeshurun" (Deut. 33:5; e.g., Ex. Rabbah 2:6, Lev. Rabbah 31:4, Num. Rabbah 15:13, *Tanhuma, Terumah* 10). Maimonides writes succinctly, "Moses was a king" (*Hilkhot Beit ha-Behirah* 6:11). But when did Moses become a king? When was the majestic crown of *malkhut*, kingship, placed squarely by the Almighty upon his head? Of course the answer is simple: it was when he stood before God on Mount Sinai. We say it every Sabbath:

> Moses rejoiced at the destiny bestowed on him when You called Your faithful servant, placing on his head a crown of glory as he stood before You on Mount Sinai; and he brought down in his hands two tablets of stone . . . (Sabbath morning *Amidah*).

Moses stood before the Almighty twice in order to receive the tablets; on which occasion was he crowned? It was when he received the second tablets; before Moses departed from Sinai, God made his face radiate, as we read, "And it came to pass when Moses came down from Mount Sinai . . . Moses did not know that the skin of his face shone" (Ex. 34:29). Only then was Moses appointed, anointed, and crowned by the Almighty.

Why was he elevated only at the second *mattan Torah* on Yom Kippur? Why was he not endowed with kingship on Shavuot, when he encountered the Almighty the first time? What happened during that destiny-charged period separating the second *mattan Torah* from the first that promoted Moses to king?

It was *shevirat ha-luhot*, the shattering of the two tablets of the testimony written with the finger of God. In other words, Moses would not have attained kingship if the tragedy of the shattering of the tablets had not taken place. Moses would have been the great prophet, the greatest of all teachers, the redeemer—but not king. What did Moses lack before the shattering of the tablets that he attained afterwards? How did this tragic and heartbreaking event enhance Moses' personality and elevate him to the heights of majesty? To answer these questions we must analyze the Jewish concept of kingship.

Power Structures

Malkhut is inseparably linked up with the human quest for companionship and co-existence. Human sociability was decreed by the Almighty at the dawn of creation, when, in His inscrutable wisdom, He proclaimed that loneliness is bad for man's growth and development—"It is not good for man to be alone" (Gen. 2:18). In order to redeem man from his tragic solitude, He created Eve to join him. Indeed, man, because of fear of loneliness, has displayed a remarkable talent for setting up social entities and linking his individual solitary life with other beings, developing thus a complex system of human relations to protect himself from the curse of being alone.

However, even if the constitution or covenant by which the group was established rests upon democratic and liberal foundations, there is no ideal equality within the group that was formed in order to help man free himself from his loneliness. No matter how progressive a particular society is, and however sincerely it strives to do away with discrimination and class distinctions, its members can never attain equality in the personal sense. Inequality within society will endure as long as man roams upon the face of the globe. The reason for this inequality lies in the paradoxical nature of man, in his individuality and uniqueness. Inequality is perhaps the shibboleth of man, his most characteristic trait, his prime mark of distinction and differentiation from the subhuman world. Our Rabbis said, "Just as people's faces are different from one another, so too are their opinions [read: personalities] different" (*Berakhot* 58a).

In every society, regardless of the social order, there are people who rule and people who are ruled; there are masters and subjects, those who instruct and those who take orders. Successful and strong man emerges on top and becomes king or ruler. The man who is frustrated, weak, or meek turns into subject. Hence, the fear of aloneness and the quest for togetherness, co-existence, and collaboration precipitated the formation of power structures and power relationships.

Let us not deceive ourselves by distinguishing between a democratic society, where personal power is limited, and a totalitarian order, which equips the ruler with absolute power. The phrase "limited power" contains an inner contradiction. Power is by its very definition absolute. When we speak of limited power, we refer to horizontal and not vertical boundaries. The area within which the individual rules is limited, but in that area the power of the individual is absolute. A judge is certainly limited in his power if seen under a horizontal aspect, but as far as judicial decisions are concerned, he wields ultimate power. He can sentence a man to death. A governor does not enjoy boundless power. Yet he has the right to pardon or commute a death sentence. The president of the United States is only the head of the executive branch of government. However, he can declare war and send many people to their deaths.

Judaism has always been very cautious in relation to political power-structures and displays little tolerance for power concentrated in the hands of an individual. Of course, we were compelled to reconcile ourselves with historical realities. No matter how imperfect government is, no matter how undesirable is the exercise of power on the part of an elected or appointed individual, anarchy is still worse. "Pray for the welfare of the government (*malkhut*)," said *Hazal*, "for without the fear of it, men would swallow one another alive" (*Avot* 3:2). Therefore Judaism reluctantly sanctioned the idea of a political community. I would categorize the attitude of the Torah vis-à-vis power-wielding by a political community as falling under the class of precepts of which *Hazal* said, "What the Torah said was aimed only at the evil inclination" (*Kiddushin* 21b).

Prerequisites of Kingship

The commandment concerning the appointment of a king is not without certain reservations. I once heard from my father zt"l that the validity of the commandment is dependent upon two prerequisites. First, there must be a historical need for the choosing of a monarch. If, for instance, a king is indispensable for the defense of the people and their land, then it is incumbent upon us to set up a monarchy. The very *baraita* that identified the verse "You shall appoint a king" (Deut. 17:15) as a positive precept speaks of two other precepts that are tightly connected with the appointment of a king: "The nation of Israel was commanded to perform three commandments upon their entrance into the Land of Israel: to appoint over themselves a king, to eradicate Amalek, and to build the Holy Temple" (*Sanhedrin* 20b). The destruction of Amalek and the construction of the

Temple are supposed to follow the appointment of a king. We must appoint a king to defend the physical and spiritual survival of the Jewish people.

Another situation which may prompt the selection of a king is anarchy and the breakdown of law and order. The Bible emphasizes, "In those days there was no king in Israel; everyone did as he pleased" (Judg. 21:25). The verse stresses this because it was exactly the determining factor which made the appointment of the king mandatory. If law and order could have prevailed without the king, there would be no need for him.

Maimonides states these two reasons in unmistakable language: "The entire purpose of appointing a king is to execute justice and to wage wars, as it is written: 'Our king shall judge us, go out before us, and wage our wars' (I Sam. 8:20)" (*Hilkhot Melakhim* 4:10). The prime reasons for appointing a king were that he would implement the principles of justice and wage war. In a word, a power structure is justified if it is created for the sake of an external goal which requires the setting up of such a structure. Only the attainment of the goal justifies the means.

There is teleology to kingship, and the purposiveness is not in the power structure itself. Each king was charged with a specific task. Each one pursued a definitive objective whose implementation was the prime reason for his ascendancy to the monarchy. David's kingdom was wholly committed to the unification of the loosely federated tribes and the complete conquest of the Land of Israel. Solomon's rule was concerned with the construction of the Temple. Hezekiah was summoned by Providence to the perpetuation of the unity of people and Torah.

The second prerequisite of kingship is that the people must request the appointment of the king. The monarch cannot be imposed on them. "And you will say, 'I will set a king over myself, like all the nations that are around me'; then you may set a king over yourself" (Deut. 17:14–15). The initiative belongs to the people, not to the *beit din*, the court. If the people do not utter such a wish, the court has no right to establish a monarchy.

"Given that the setting up of a king was a commandment, why did the Holy One look with disfavor upon the request made by the people of Samuel for a king?" asks Maimonides (*Hilkhot Melakhim* 1:2). He explains that "It was because the people asked in a querulous spirit. Their request was prompted not by the desire to fulfill a precept but by a desire to rid themselves of Samuel the prophet, as it is written, 'For they have not rejected you but they have rejected Me' (I Sam. 8:7)."

But why should the way in which the request was made affect the validity or the binding character of the mitzvah? Let us assume that the request was not phrased in proper and intelligent language and that the motive was the wrong one. There was still no reason for God and Samuel to look with disfavor upon something which constitutes a basic precept, a biblical commandment. The wrong motivation does not nullify the worth of a mitzvah; a false approach must not render null and void a deserving, noble act.

The only logical conclusion to be derived from Maimonides is that the request for a king is of central significance because it is the source of the norm. It legitimizes the power structure created by the appointment. Since the request is a *conditio sine qua non* for the fulfillment or implementation of the commandment of appointing a king, it is necessary that the request be formulated in compliance with the Halakhah. And if the request is not phrased in the proper halakhic terms and is motivated by the wrong desires, then it fails to produce results and is not binding. Whenever the appointment of a king is not mandatory or obligatory, it is sinful.

Reluctance to Establish Power Structures

The reason for the reluctance on the part of Judaism to set up permanent power structures such as a monarchy is due to two motives. First, as Lord Acton said, "Power tends to corrupt;

absolute power corrupts absolutely." The greatest of all rulers, the most ideal, charismatic leader, is bound willy-nilly to step over the boundary line of legitimate authority and engage in some kind of tyranny, in arbitrary decisions and unfair practices.

Second, man in general is unfit to rule. He has no right to exercise dominion over his fellow man. Certainly, Judaism says, the ruler may be capable; otherwise he would not be a ruler. He may be brilliant. God may have blessed him with a sense of leadership and an inspiring personality. Certainly those who are subordinate may be dull, meek, and in need of guidance. Yet, Judaism asks, does intellectual superiority justify the exercise of power? Do personal traits, no matter how relevant, grant a person the right to order, instruct, and dominate?

Judaism has never measured the worth of a human personality by the yardstick of the creative talents with which the individual is blessed. A contrite heart is more cherished by the Almighty than a keen mind. A modest and humble person—even if he lags behind others intellectually because circumstances prevent him from actualizing the human potential which God implanted in him—is more acceptable to God than a vain and proud person who is favored with the opportunity to achieve fame and take advantage of every talent God has vested in him.

Man has not been invited to share in the attributes of *melukhah* and *memshalah*, kingdom and power, which belong exclusively to the Eternal One. True, the Almighty quite often asks man to join Him and, paradoxically, to be like Him, to "walk in His ways" (Deut. 28:9). "Just as He is gracious and merciful, so you shall be gracious and merciful" (*Shabbat* 133b). Yet power is an exception to this rule. Power is an exclusively divine potency to which man has no access. *Melekh Elyon* dislikes *melekh evyon* if the latter begins to take himself seriously. The quest for power precipitated the oldest sin on the part of mankind. The serpent took advantage of the human urge to rule, to be mighty, to dominate, to emerge victorious from every engagement, to legislate his own laws. The snake told Eve that by eating of the Tree of Knowledge she would realize her ambition. She would become powerful, "and you shall be like God, knowing good and evil" (Gen. 3:5).

Judaism, therefore, has always been confronted with an antinomy implied in the very core of the exercise of power, including the judicial power structure. On the one hand, it is convinced that due to the human situation, one cannot dispense with these structures; on the other hand, it has consistently argued that man is not entitled to sit in judgment over his fellow man. Only God has the right to judge people. "God stands in the divine assembly; among the judges He pronounces judgment" (Ps. 82:1). That is why Judaism complicated the judicial procedures and almost eliminated not only bodily punishment—execution and lashes—but also monetary fines, *kenassot*. Nowadays, we cannot impose *kenassot*, because we lack the authority of *semikhah* (*Hilkhot Sanhedrin* 5:8–9).

Even as regards trivial everyday litigation in civil matters, Judaism, with fear and foreboding, warns the *dayyan*, the justice who is authorized to resolve the controversy, that he is engaged in something awesome and dreadful. If he should err or, alas, even falter in the execution of justice, his sin will be unpardonable.

> At all times a judge should think of himself as if a sword were suspended over his head and Gehenna gaping under him. He should know whom he is judging and before Whom he is judging, and Who will call him to account if he deviates from the line of truth, as it is written (Ps. 82:1), "God stands in the divine assembly; among the judges He pronounces judgment," and it is also written (II Chr. 19:6), "Consider what you are doing; for you judge not on behalf of man, but on behalf of the Lord" (*Hilkhot Sanhedrin* 23:8).

Malkhut *as a Metaphysical Idea*

Malkhut signifies not only a concrete power structure, political institution, or political community—such as a kingdom, government, or state—but also a great metaphysical idea, a glorious vision which the covenantal community has beheld and with which it has been fascinated since the dawn of its millennial history. *Malkhut* as a metaphysical idea turns into a great ethical norm which aims to achieve the ultimate objective in Judaism.

Within the metaphysical frame of reference, *malkhut* is not the prerogative or exclusive possession of one individual, clan, or dynasty. It was bestowed upon man in general on that mysterious Friday when God fashioned him out of dust and made him an individual, a being, unique and singular, for whom there is no substitute. Later, man lost *malkhut* when he sinned, and God wants His covenantal community to restore the quality of *malkhut* to its members. The potential of *malkhut* is implanted in every Jew: "All Jews are the children of kings" (*Bava Metzia* 113b).

How does *malkhut* as a moral-metaphysical idea express itself? Again, we must consult the Halakhah. We stated above that when there is an urgent need for such an institution, it is incumbent upon us to appoint a king. The political power structure is thus of a teleological nature; it is significant whenever history burdens it with a specific mission. In a word, *malkhut* equals the awareness that one has an assignment to carry out. The equation is, of course, reversible. We may say that assignment-awareness equals *malkhut*. In a metaphysical sense, the king is he who feels committed to the achievement of a great goal, the realization of an objective.

The king carries a burden. In Hebrew, *massa*, a burden, is to be understood in the physical sense and also in the spiritual sense. *Massa* also means prophecy: "The Babylonian *massa*, a prophecy of Isaiah son of Amoz" (Isa. 13:1); "*Massa*, the word of the Lord concerning Israel" (Zech. 12:1). The prophet is burdened. He is dedicated, committed; he is not free. *Malkhut* takes away freedom—but the taking away of freedom enhances one's personality.

Here we encounter Judaism's doctrine of assignment. Each person was created in order to carry out a certain task. Each individual is entrusted with a specific assignment, which he must implement no matter how difficult or embarrassing. It is not coincidental that in Hebrew we do not distinguish between wage and reward, between contracted and noncontracted compensation, the way we do in other languages. In English, a wage means the pay a laborer receives for performing a certain task; a reward means a generous gift where there is no obligation or commitment to offer a payment. In Biblical and Talmudic Hebrew, the noun *sakhar* has the connotation of reward as well as wage. Judaism apparently considers the good bestowed upon man for a meritorious life as an earned wage, not as a gratuitous reward. Man is under a contractual obligation to his employer—who happens to be the Almighty. Man is actually a hireling who is contracted to perform a specific task; upon completing his assignment he may lay claim to well-earned compensation.

> Man's days are determined; You know the number of his months, and You have set him limits that he cannot pass. [Therefore,] turn away from him, that he may be at ease, until he shall accomplish, as a hireling, his day (Job 14:5–6).

The life of man is like a day which has been completed by the hireling; he has been appointed to fulfill an assignment.

The doctrine of assignment is spelled out in unmistakable terms in the Book of Esther.

> Think not that you shall escape in the king's house, more than all the Jews. For if you altogether hold your peace

at this time, then will relief and deliverance arise to the Jews from another place, but you and your father's house will perish; and who knows whether you are not come to royal estate for such a time as this (Esth. 4:13–14).

The doctrine of assignment consists of three basic component parts, all of them spelled out by Mordecai. First, each individual is assigned a task which he must implement, and which does not transcend his ability. The mission of saving the people was once placed squarely upon the strong shoulders of David and his commander-in-chief, Joab. And now the same mission was placed upon the frail shoulders of a delicate and lonely young woman who steadily lived in the shadow of rejection and death. She was burdened with a gigantic task. She was a queen not because Ahasuerus crowned her but on account of the great assignment entrusted to her.

Second, even in the face of human failure, betrayal, or indifference, God's will nonetheless will be done. The assignment will be carried out—if not by the assigned individual, then by someone else. "For if you altogether hold your peace at this time, then will relief and deliverance arise to the Jews from another place" (Esth. 4:14). Third, the individual who does not answer the call of history, does not respond to the challenge, does not carry out his assignment—such a person is a traitor and his sin is unpardonable. "But you and your father's house will perish" (Esth. 4:14).

Open Existence — Present, "with vs" accessible, welcoming

Malkhut contains another dimension, namely, that of an open existence. Let us explain it by introducing the kabbalistic term *Shekhinah*. This refers to the ubiquitous presence of God within the world, within the natural cosmic drama. When we mention *E-l*, we refer to God in His remoteness and transcendence beyond the fringes of the universe. He is "*E-l mistater*, the hidden God" (Isa. 48:15). However, when we say *Shekhinah,* we address ourselves to the One who has never been distant from us, who stands next to us, who trails behind us and walks in front of us, who is "your shadow, on your right hand" (Ps. 121:5). *Shekhinah* is the God with whom we converse, to whom we pray and cling in times of distress, to whom we sing a hymn of praise when destiny is good to us, in whom we confide and in whom we find comfort and solace. In short, *Shekhinah* denotes an open and communicative Divine Presence, a nearness which spans the gap separating Creator from creature. The verb *shin-khaf-nun* means to abide, to be present, to reside.

However, the term *Shekhinah* signifies immanence and proximity not only in a communicative sense but also in a sympathetic sense. *Shekhinah* is the mother who is kind and understanding, who displays unlimited tolerance and patience for her imperfect child, forgiving his shortcomings, overlooking his errors, and not minding his nonsensical insolence. Patiently she waits for her child to come back, to regret, to confess, and to amend his ways. She never deserts her child; she never deserts the sinner.

In a word, *Shekhinah* not only communicates with man from the twinkle of the star or the flight of the bird or from the depths of his personality, but also has compassion for man. She shares his trouble, his cares, his tragic experiences and failures for which he himself is responsible. "When a man suffers, what does the *Shekhinah* say? 'I am burdened by My head; I am burdened by My arm'" (*Hagigah* 15b, *Sanhedrin* 46a).

The same applies to the individual who wants to achieve kingship. The Kabbalah equates *Shekhinah* with *malkhut.* An open existence is a royal existence. The king resides in the midst of the people; he is always close to his subjects and accessible to them. Everybody and everyone may approach the king—widow, orphan, woodchopper, water-drawer, vagabond, stranger, old-timer, sinner, or thief. Each may complain to him, demand justice, and ask for help. "Then came there two women

that were harlots unto the king and stood before him" (I Kings
3:16). "And as the king of Israel was passing by upon the wall,
there cried a woman unto him, saying, 'Help, my lord, my king'"
(II Kings 6:26). Such absurd rules about which we read in the
Megillah—"that whoever enters the inner court without having
received an invitation from the king, there is one law for him,
that he be put to death" (Esth. 4:11)—do not exist in the annals
of Judaism. Anybody could knock on the door of the Jewish king
and come in. That is because anybody can knock on the door of
the King of kings and come in!

In a word, man who aspires to kingship must open up his
existence; he must be communicative, accessible, and capable of
coordinating his basic needs with the needs of others. When we
say an open existence, we do not mean the cultivation of gre-
gariousness or sociability. These are not necessarily the traits of
existential openness; an open existence can be achieved even by
the introvert or the introspective personality. What we want to
express through this term is that man, while living, working,
suffering, rejoicing, and moving along an endless trail of his
own which no one else will ever cross, must always remember
that, in spite of the fact that he is a singular being, he is not a
single being. God's concern encompasses not only him but
countless individuals like him who also wander, each one along
his own trail, each burdened with his own problems and cares,
traveling toward an unknown destiny.

Malkhut, in general historical terms, precipitates the separation of the king from his people, his elevation over them, and
his existential exclusiveness. However, in Judaism, *malkhut*
means integration of the individual in the community and existential all-inclusiveness and openness. Whether *klal Yisrael*
consists of sinners or saints, we must accept it as it is and open
up our existence to all. Any act of separating people, of creating
a sectarian philosophy, of promoting and cultivating isolation-
ism and moral religious egocentrism and self-righteousness—
such an act violates the principle of existential openness!

The king opens himself up to everyone and embraces the entire nation, without excluding anybody. The king's existential openness is of both a communicative and a sympathetic nature. Maimonides writes of the king, "his heart is the heart of the entire congregation of Israel" (*Hilkhot Melakhim* 3:6); the heart of the king is the heart of the people. *Malkhut* requires of man not only to be aware of the existence of others, but also to feel, to experience their existence as if it were his own. In other words, *malkhut* requires of man to join and fit together concerns, wishes, dreams, and, particularly, travails and suffering.

As long as one is cognizant of the existence of others, one is categorized as a *re'a*, an acquaintance or neighbor. But the very instant that one begins to perceive another—not just to know him but to feel his existence, experience his joys and frustrations, agonies and hopes—one turns from a *re'a* into an *ah*, a brother. This is a higher degree of co-existence, of interrelatedness and companionship.

Brothers are united by existential bonds—one destiny, one memory. The precepts of *tzedakah* and *gemilut hasadim* are nurtured by the doctrine of the sympathetic, brotherly, open existence. In speaking of *tzedakah*, the Torah constantly employs the term *ah*, not *re'a*: "If your brother becomes impoverished" (Lev. 25:25, 35, 39); "If there shall be a destitute person among you, one of your brothers" (Deut. 15:7).

On the other hand, when the Torah speaks about civil law—not to inflict harm on someone—it employs the term *re'a*. "Do not covet the house of *re'ekha*" (Ex. 20:14). "Do not move the landmark of *re'akha*" (Deut. 19:14). The fact that he is my neighbor imposes a duty and an obligation upon me. I should respect his property and his rights; I must not inflict any harm or damage on him. But this does not entitle the *re'a* to my support—that I should share his troubles and be helpful to him in times of need. For that, the bond of *re'a* is too weak. You need a stronger bond—that of *ah,* a brother!

Maimonides emphasized the element of brotherliness in conjunction with *tzedakah*: "All Jews and those attached to them are like brothers, as it is said, 'You are sons to the Lord your God' (Deut. 14:1); and if a brother does not show mercy to his brother, then who will have mercy on him?" (*Hilkhot Matenot Aniyim* 10:2). One is obligated to help the unfortunate and to share his woes and misery. Halakhically, *tzedakah* does not consist exclusively of extending material help. Sharing experiences and displaying sympathy and compassion is part of the mitzvah of *tzedakah*. At times, it is more relevant and more important than the material help we extend to someone else.

The Authority of the Teacher

At this juncture, a new concept of power emerges. We said before that the Torah was very reluctant about sanctioning and promoting unlimited power. It simply reconciled itself with historical realities. But there is one form of power or authority which was sanctioned wholeheartedly: the authority exercised by the teacher vis-à-vis his pupil.

The commanding influence of the master over his disciple was accepted by the Torah without any qualifications or reservations. In fact, spiritual authority is quite often superior to political power. It endures longer and is more inclusive. At times, spiritual authority borders on the ultimate, on blind obedience. (Of course, the teacher should be an ideal one; this kind of power can be misused and abused by unscrupulous teachers.)

For instance, the impact that the Baal Shem Tov had upon his disciples—and through them on the lives of thousands of Jews throughout two centuries—can hardly be matched by any ruler in the history of the political community. The same is true of the Gaon of Vilna. The latter was a contemporary of Napoleon (though older by several decades). Napoleon is considered by many historians to have personified the prototype of the man of power, the charismatic leader, warlord, legislator, and king. Yet the Gaon's posthumous authority outlived that of Napoleon and many others.

While Judaism is perturbed about political power and tries to limit its exercise as much as possible, it encourages the disciple to give boundless respect to his teacher, to listen to him and try to fulfill his teacher's wishes. The word *et* in the verse "You shall revere *et* the Lord Your God" (Deut. 6:13) indicates the inclusion of Torah scholars (*Pesahim* 22b). God is not ready to share His authority and power with kings or the political community. However, He is willing to share his authority and power within the spiritual community, with the teacher.

Two reasons lie at the root of the Judaic glorification and idealization of the teacher, the *rav* or *rebbi*. First, the authority of the *rebbi* is not imposed upon the pupil, the *talmid*. No political instrument is used; no coercive action is undertaken to foist the authority of the *rav* upon the pupil. The pupil of his own free will yields to the authority of the teacher. At times, the teacher feels embarrassed by the pupil's deference. While the political authority of the king is nurtured by fear, the spiritual authority of the teacher is rooted in deep affection and respect. The teacher is a master; but the mastery of the teacher is blessed by the Almighty, who Himself is the teacher par excellence. The teacher's mastery is expressed in Halakhah: "All tasks that a slave performs for his master, a disciple performs for his master" (*Ketubbot* 96a). However, it is mastery which does not result in slavery but in self-redemption and freedom.

The second reason Judaism glorifies the teacher and idealizes him is that authority and ownership are identical concepts. Authority is vested in the owner, who can dispose of or use his property in any arbitrary fashion he chooses. The head of the political community is denied authority because he does not own his so-called subjects. They are his equals, over whom he has no right to rule. It is God's authority that is boundless, because He is the Maker of all things. "The earth is the Lord's and the fullness thereof, the world and they who dwell in it; for

He has founded it upon the seas . . . Lift up your heads, O gates . . . and the King of glory shall come in!" (Ps. 24:1–2, 7). He is the King of unlimited authority, *Melekh ha-kavod*, because He is the creator. *Melekh evyon* has no authority, since he is no creator.

But if the teacher is not a creator *ex nihilo*, Judaism looks upon him at least as a fashioner, an artisan who takes primordial matter and impresses form upon it. The teacher shapes something amorphous into something beautiful and fascinating. The subject does not belong to the king, but the pupil belongs to the teacher, because the latter trained and enlightened his mind, sensitized his heart, molded his personality, and brought out the noblest and finest in him.

Judaism considers the teaching of Torah a reflection of the infinite process of creation initiated by God at the dawn of existence, which has never come to a close. God summons man to participate in the great, wondrous drama of creation. The teacher, the *rebbi*, answers the call and joins the Creator; hence, he has a share in the student. He owns him because he is responsible for that for which the student stands. And it is self-evident that with the ownership comes authority.

Abraham and Sarah participated in this creative gesture because they taught and enlightened people. "And the souls that they had made in Haran" (Gen. 12:5): how can one make a soul? Only God can create a soul! The Midrash answers: "This teaches that Abraham converted the men and Sarah converted the women" (Gen. Rabbah 39:14). Their spiritual authority was sanctioned by God.

The creative gesture of teaching consists in the opening up of one's existence. It consists not in the mechanical passing on of information, but in letting the student share in the great spiritual treasures stored up in the depths and recesses of the teacher's personality. One cannot teach unless one tears down all the barriers separating individuals from each other, unless one is ready to establish an existential community where there

Teaching as Communion

DL.: Not in the reality!!
Truly! Larger than life! Define w/ Distance

is an exchange of ideas, a continuous flow of thought, a conflu-
ence of experiences, one rhythm of heartbeats, compassion, and
affection.

In the master-disciple relationship, *malkhut* finds its realization. No wonder *Hazal* spoke of rabbis as *melakhim* (*Gittin*
62a). The rabbis were kings, but they were not wealthy. We
know of the poverty in which our scholars found themselves.
They were *melakhim* because God delegated them authority—
authority which not even kings possessed. To be a disciple
means to participate in the existential experience of the master.
To be a teacher means to open up the recesses of one's own existence.

The glorious tradition of the dynasty of the House of David,
which is supposed to find its culmination in the King Messiah,
rests upon the king-teacher doctrine. Is the Messiah a politically powerful monarch who will foist his authority upon mankind
by using the sword? Certainly not! Rather, the Messiah is the
great, wondrous teacher-prophet, who will instruct and enlight-
en, and by so doing he will redeem the world. Maimonides
writes:

> Because the king who will arise from the seed of David
> will possess more wisdom than Solomon and will be a
> great prophet, approaching Moses our teacher, he will
> teach the whole of the Jewish people and instruct them
> in the way of God; and all nations will come to hear him,
> as it is said (Isa. 2:2–3): "And at the end of days it shall
> come to pass that the mount of the Lord's house shall be
> established as the top of the mountains [and peoples
> shall flow unto it, and many nations shall go and say:
> Come you and let us go up to the mountain of the Lord,
> to the house of the God of Jacob, and He will teach us of
> His ways and we will walk in His paths]" (*Hilkhot
> Teshuvah* 9:2).

Malkhut thus achieves its complete realization in the teacher-king union. It has absolutely nothing in common with the Platonic philosopher-king. Moses was the greatest king in our history. Why? Because he was the greatest teacher the Jews ever had.

Facing Defeat

Yet no matter how exalted the idea of *malkhut* is—and exalted it is indeed—it must be dovetailed with another idea, namely, that of *kedushah*, sanctity. Of course, *malkhut* when realized is a grand experience. A closed-up, fenced-in, self-oriented, ego-conscious, and "within-minded" individual opens up toward the outside, tears down all fences, changes his orientation, and, with a gesture of magnanimity, spreads out his arms to embrace God's world, inviting everybody to share with him all the goods he possesses, all the treasures he has jealously stocked away. Nevertheless, the king must assume another commitment, *kedushah*, if his *malkhut* is to reach perfection, if dominion is to change into service, fear into love, and obedience into a great ecstasy, thus converting the political community into a spiritual-metaphysical community.

To acquire the synthesis of *kedushah* and *malkhut*, the king must be aware of his assignment. He must try to meet the challenge of history, to answer the summons of the historical hour. He opens up his existence and tears down all the barriers. He sheds his selfishness and egocentrism. He understands everybody and sympathizes with them. He is a great teacher who continues on, even in the face of failure.

Until the Golden Calf episode, Moses had never failed. He was victorious until that time in all his undertakings. He was the messenger of fulfillment, the angel of realization; his message consisted of joyous words for which the Jews were longing, "I have surely remembered you" (Ex. 3:16). Of course, every promise of God will be fulfilled; every pledge will be implemented. But one has to wait. This was the destiny of Abraham;

but Moses' destiny was different. God revealed Himself to Moses through the medium of the Tetragrammaton, which indicates immediate realization and complete victory over the causal nexus of historical events.

Moses was the fortunate one who prophesied divine openness and revelation, who brought with him the message of victory, whose authority was not questioned. The pillar of fire, of triumph, was marching in front of him, and the clouds of protection and safety behind him.

Victory and *malkhut*, in the opinion of Judaism, are two contradictory and mutually exclusive concepts in this world. As long as man is always victorious, as long as he is always triumphant, as long as his endeavors are blessed with success continually, as long as he continues to surge ahead without being stopped and made to retreat—he cannot attain *malkhut* interwoven with *kedushah*.

In order to be qualified to receive the crown of light (not from man but from the Almighty), to attain the pinnacle of *malkhut* and *kedushah*, one must lose at least one major battle; one must be crushed and defeated, one's aspirations a shamble, one's dreams, visions, and hopes a heap of ashes. In order to rise from that heap of ashes and dust and ascend the throne of majesty and kingship, we must emulate Moses. Moses could not achieve *malkhut* as long as his course to greatness was continuous ascent, without alterations, angles, or curves. When all his aspirations were coming true, when his hopes seemed to be in the process of realization, when his visions appeared to turn into realities—Moses could not attain the pinnacle of *malkhut*.

Moses was appointed king only when the voice of God declared, "Get you down, for the people have dealt corruptly" (Ex. 32:7), only when he was thrust back from his heroically conquered exalted positions and points of vantage, only when he realized that he had failed miserably and the people he had brought out of Egypt were not ready to receive the Torah, only when, in black despair and desolation, he threw down the tablets and broke them, only when he was rejected by God and deflated completely.

It is God's will that man should not achieve that which he is meant to achieve without being once defeated, without failing and losing his existential security, without relapsing to lower ontological levels, without experiencing *hester panim* (what the mystics of the Middle Ages called "the dark night of the soul"), without finding himself in front of the tightly closed gates of heaven and hearing the echo of his own voice coming back from dark, uncharted spaces. The breaking of the tablets is an integral part of human destiny. God decreed man to fail when He addressed Himself to Adam and told him, "Thorns also and thistles shall it bring forth to you. . . . By the sweat of your brow shall you eat bread, until you return unto the ground" (Gen. 3:18–19).

Everybody, great or small, is subject to God's dictum; none can escape. No one can acquire greatness—not even Moses, the greatest and most glorious of all teachers—without experiencing defeat and failure.

Judaism taught man how to accept failure and not get lost—not only how to be defeated and not disintegrate, not only how to be crushed and not be overcome with despair and resignation, but also how to rise after one has fallen, how to pick oneself up without help after one has been thrown from the top of the mountain into the abyss.

Judaism taught man how to assemble patiently the debris of the shattered tablets and restore their original integrity, or how to hew new tablets from the hard rock and climb the steep mount, rising above a black and gaping precipice alone, how to retrace one's steps up the mountain along its winding and curving paths, how to wait for the Almighty, even though He is sometimes slow in joining man.

"Carve two stone tablets like the first ones, and I shall write upon these tablets the words that were on the first tablets, which you did break; and be ready in the morning, and ascend

Mount Sinai in the morning, and present yourself there to Me on the top of the mountain" (Ex. 34:1–2). It is difficult to do things all over again; it is hard to repeat something in which we have just failed. It is almost impossible to believe that this time we shall succeed while we failed yesterday in the same endeavor. And yet, nevertheless, "Carve two stone tablets . . . and ascend Mount Sinai in the morning." This is our assignment, this is our destiny. And at this juncture, *malkut* and *kedushah* meet.

❧ The Inversion of Jewish History

Inverted Letters

Preceding and following two consecutive verses in *Parashat Beha'alotekha*, we find an inverted Hebrew letter *nun*:

> And it came to pass, when the ark set forward, that Moses said, "Arise, O Lord, and let Your enemies be scattered, and let Your foes flee before You." And when it came to rest, he said, "Return, O Lord, unto the ten thousand thousands of Israel" (Num. 10:35–36).

The nuns emphasize, say *Hazal* (*Shabbat* 116a), that the two verses are out of context. For example, it would seem that the verses could have been beautifully inserted in context at the end of *Pekudei*:

> For God's cloud was on the tabernacle by day, and fire was in the cloud by night, before the eyes of all the house of Israel at each stage of their journey (Ex. 40:38).

Why, then, would the Torah insert the verses into a section within which they would stand out as out of context? The Torah is always careful about connectivity, development, and transition in its narratives. What is the thread of connectivity between the themes the Torah develops in *Parashat Beha'alotekha?* In fact, as we read the various narratives, we seem to be jumping like a bee on a clear, warm summer morning from flower to flower, accumulating the sweet nectar.

The *parashah* commences with the sanctification of the Levites. (The several verses dedicated to the *menorah* actually belong in *Parashat Naso,* as Rashi [Num. 8:2, s.v. *beha'alotekha*] suggests when he says, "When Aaron saw the offerings of the princes, he became upset.") Then the Torah tells us about the Passover of the second year in the desert, and then about Pesah Sheni, the paschal sacrifice offered in Iyar by one who was far away or impure during the first Pesah in Nissan. Following the description of Pesah Sheni, we have, without any transition, a description of the pillar of cloud guiding the people on their journeys. "Whenever the cloud lifted from over the tent, then the Israelites would set out" (Num. 9:17).

Following the narrative about the cloud, the Torah relates the commandment pertaining to the *hatzotzerot,* the two trumpets used to assemble the community and signal when the camps were to journey. At the conclusion of the section dealing with the trumpets, the Torah reviews the previous theme and presents the details of the order in which the camps traveled: Judah at the head, followed by Issachar, and so forth. Then, after the Torah describes the organization of the camps and how they moved and traveled, suddenly we hear a conversation between Moses and his father-in-law which, *prima facie,* is puzzling and enigmatic.

> Moses said unto Hobab the son of Reuel the Midianite, Moses' father-in-law: "We are journeying unto the place of which the Lord said: 'I will give it you'; come with us,

and we will do good to you; for the Lord has spoken good concerning Israel." And he said unto him: "I will not go; but I will depart to my own land, and to my kindred." And he said: "Leave us not, I pray you; forasmuch as you know how we are to encamp in the wilderness, and you shall be as eyes for us. And it shall be, if you go with us, that whatever good the Lord shall do unto us, the same will we do unto you" (Num. 10:29–32).

Following this conversation, we are suddenly confronted with the *parashah* bracketed by the inverted *nuns*. The letters are inverted because what follows is a story which inverted our historical process. Alas, the *parashah* is really one sad tale which changes Jewish history completely, from top to bottom.

The Final Journey

Let us go back to the Exodus. When the Almighty charged Moses with the assignment of redeeming the Jews, liberating them from Egypt, he told him, "It shall be your sign that it was I who sent you: when you have freed the people from Egypt, you shall worship the Lord on this mountain" (Ex. 3:12).

In other words, the Almighty told Moses that the Exodus drama would not be consummated until they had worshipped God at this mountain. The worship centered around the *Mishkan,* the Tabernacle. In fact, the very day after Moses came down from Mount Sinai, he assembled the people and told them that a Tabernacle was to be constructed, and Bezalel began work. It is no wonder that following the Decalogue in *Parashat Yitro,* God mentioned to Moses the construction of an altar:

Make for Me an altar of earth. . . . And if you make Me an altar of stone, you shall not build it of hewn stones; for if you lift up your tool upon it, you have profaned it. Neither shall you go up by steps unto My altar, that your nakedness be not exposed upon it (Ex. 20:21–23).

Had the Jews not succumbed to the hysteria of the masses, had they not constructed the Golden Calf, the two objectives would have been realized much sooner. Because of their sin, the schedule was changed and the realization of "You shall worship the Lord on this mountain" was delayed. If the calf had not been made and the whole tragedy had thus been avoided, Moses would have come down on the seventeenth of Tammuz and immediately they would have started to construct the Tabernacle. Because of the sin, Moses had to spend eighty more days on Mount Sinai in prayer. He came down from Mount Sinai on the day following Yom Kippur. After this delay of eighty days, after Moses came down with the second set of tablets and the message of forgiveness, he quickly assembled the congregation and told them about the immediate task to be discharged—the building of the Tabernacle. The Tabernacle was completed and put together on the first of Nissan, which, according to our Rabbis (*Sifra Shemini, Parashah* 1; Rashi Lev. 9:1), was the eighth day of consecration, *millu'im*, the day on which the princes began to offer their gifts to the Tabernacle. When the giving of the Torah and the construction of the Tabernacle were achieved, the redemption found its realization. "You shall worship the Lord on this mountain" was translated into reality. There was no purpose in extending the sojourn any longer.

The Torah in *Naso* tells us about the final act in the dedication of the Tabernacle, namely, the sacrifices by the princes. The Torah does not fail to mention a secondary matter like the sanctification of the Levites. The Torah apprises us in *Tzav* about the sanctification of the *kohanim*, priests, which was of primary significance. In a word, with the dedication of the Tabernacle by the princes and the election of the Levites, everything which was necessary in order to have the Tabernacle serve the great purpose of worship was prepared and ready; the work was completed.

They were ready to march on the thirteenth of Nissan. However, the cloud did not move or rise, because on the next day

the paschal sacrifice was to be offered. So the march was postponed until after Passover. Everybody knew that the stay of the
Jews in the wilderness of Sinai was coming to a close and the
march would resume after they offered the paschal sacrifice.
The Torah tells us about the paschal sacrifice in *Beha'alotekha*,
because it was the only obstacle to the resumption of the march.
The Torah also tells us about the sanctification of the Levites in
the context of the final preparations. (It was not as important as
the sanctification of the priests, which is why the Torah tells us
about the sanctification of the priests in *Tzav* and *Tetzaveh*. One
could operate the Tabernacle without the Levites; their main
function was *shir,* song.) Thus the two prerequisites for moving
on to the Promised Land—the giving of the Torah and the construction of the Tabernacle—were finally fulfilled. All four free-
doms were attained, "I will take out . . . I will save . . . I will
redeem . . . I will take . . ." The hour was struck for the fifth freedom to be realized and be translated into a reality: "I will bring
you into the land" (Ex. 6:6–8).

The march was supposed to last several days; that is why
the Torah reveals to us the details of the march. First, the pillar of cloud was the guide, an instrument in the hands of the
Almighty (Num. 9:22–23). The Torah then tells us how the
camps were arranged for marching, which tribes formed the
avant-garde and which formed the rear guard. The Torah
speaks of *tziv'otam,* that is, their hosts of warriors. In this context, the Torah also relates to us the story of the two trumpets
because the signal system was very important. Moses had to
instruct the various camps on their march to the Promised
Land, so there need for communication—the two silver
trumpets.

> When both [trumpets] are blown, the whole congregation
> shall assemble before you at the entrance of the tent of
> meeting. But if only one is blown, then the leaders, the
> heads of the tribes of Israel, shall assemble before you.

When you blow a *teru'ah*, the camps on the east side shall set out; when you blow a second *teru'ah*, the camps on the south side shall set out. A *teru'ah* is to be blown whenever they are to set out (Num. 10.3–6).

Expectation and tension permeate the pages of *Beha'alotekha*. There is a mood of mobilization and rigid order. All the conditions have been met, the reward is about to be granted, the promise to Abraham is finally about to be fulfilled. The people are on their final triumphal march. "In the second year, in the second month, on the twentieth day of the month, the cloud lifted from over the tabernacle of the covenant. Then the Israelites set out on their journey" (Num. 10:11–12). It was not one of the many journeys; it was *the* journey, the final journey.

"Come with Us and We Will Do Good to You"

Interesting is the conversation between Moses and his father-in-law. We get a glimpse into Moses, into his mood during the days after the second Passover, as the people begin to march. He speaks in a climate of serenity, of peace of mind, of unqualified assurance. He expects great things as he speaks of the final journey to the Promised Land. No delays, no procrastination— it is going to happen right now, not tomorrow. Sometimes I want to cry when I read this *parashah*. Look at the simplicity with which the great Moses, the master of all wise men and the father of all prophets, speaks. He uses the grammatical first person: "We are journeying . . . come with us, and we will do good to you; for the Lord has spoken good concerning Israel" (Num. 10:29). There is enough *hesed* and goodness and happiness to be transmitted to others and to be shared with them. Join our triumphal march toward our destiny, Moses says to Jethro; it may become your destiny as well. This was not an invitation extended by an individual to his father-in-law. Moses spoke as a representative of *Kenesset Yisrael* inviting every generation of converts to join in the march, provided they subject themselves to the same divine discipline required of the Jewish people.

Moses was certain—there was not even a shadow of doubt in his mind—that he was going to enter the Promised Land. He and the entire congregation would be classified not only as *yotze'ei Mitzrayim*, those who departed from Egypt, but as *ba'ei ha-aretz,* those who come into the Land. He was convinced that he would see the beautiful land, the hills of Judea, the prairie land of the Sharon Valley, the mount of Lebanon. Later he would pray, though his prayer did not come true: "Let me cross over to see the good land beyond the Jordan, that good hill country and the Lebanon" (Deut. 3:25). But at this time he felt no need for prayer; there was no doubt about his destiny.

The whole operation, if successfully brought to a close, would have lasted several days. And at that time, there was no need for spies and scouts to explore the land, to see whether the land was good or bad, whether the cities were walled or open, whether the population there was strong or weak, healthy or sickly. Intelligence work is necessary only if one has doubts. This was the pre-doubt period in Jewish history.

The *parashah* of "*Vayehi bi-nesoa ha-aron*" did not seem misplaced before the great reversal took place, before the Jews alienated God, before they fell from Him, before they had doubts and sent the spies. Indeed, it was the continuation of the great story of the final, triumphal messianic march into the Land of Israel, which was supposed to take place approximately 3,500 years ago.

> And they set forward from the mount of the Lord three days' journey; and the ark of the covenant of the Lord went before them three days' journey, to seek out a resting-place for them. And the cloud of the Lord was over them by day, when they set forward from the camp. And it came to pass, when the ark set forward [leading them

into the Land of Israel], that Moses said, "Arise, O Lord, and let Your enemies be scattered, and let Your foes flee before You." And when it came to rest, he said, "Return, O Lord, unto the ten thousand thousands of Israel" (Num. 10:33–36).

There would have been no need for an inverted *nun* at the beginning and an inverted *nun* at the end. The verse would have been the climax of the whole story, not an inversion. Jewish history would have taken a different course. Had Moses entered the Land of Israel, our history would never have been taken from us. The messianic era would have commenced with the conquest of the Land of Israel by Moses.

The Graves of Desire

Moses believed with a great passion and love that the final march of redemption had begun. But suddenly something happened. "And the mixed multitude that was among them fell to lusting; and the children of Israel also wept, saying: 'Would that we were given flesh to eat!' " (Num. 11:4).

Moses had gone through many crises. He had lived through many distressful experiences and moments. Worst of all was the Golden Calf, which threatened to terminate the very relationship between God and Israel. Yet he never panicked, never complained, never acted out of black despair. On the contrary, steadfastly and heroically, he petitioned the Almighty for forgiveness, defending the people, arguing their case like an attorney in court. Our Rabbis describe this by way of a metaphor, emphasizing the element of strength and boldness. "Moses took hold of the Holy One, blessed be He, like a man who seizes his fellow by his garment, and he said to Him: Sovereign of the Universe, I will not let You go until You forgive and pardon them" (*Berakhot* 32a). Yet in *Beha'alotekha*, instead of defending the people, Moses began to complain, almost accusing them.

> And Moses said to the Lord, "Why have you dealt ill with Your servant? Why have I not found favor in Your sight, that You lay the burden of all this people upon me? Did I conceive this people, did I bear them, that You should say to me: Carry them in your bosom, as a nurse carries a suckling, to the land that You did swear to their fathers?" (Num. 11:11–12).

We hear the echo of the complaint Moses uttered when his first mission to Pharaoh ended in failure: "Why have You sent me?" (Ex. 5:22). That is the question of an inexperienced man, not of a leader who has taken his people out of Egypt. Why did Moses now feel discouraged? Why didn't he offer prayers for the people, as was his practice in earlier situations of this kind? The people had committed no murder, no sexual promiscuity, no robbery—they were just overcome by desire and they wept. They did not yell or throw stones at Moses as they did in other situations. They were not threatening anyone. They simply desired, a fact enshrined in the name given to the place, Kivrot ha-Ta'avah. This name could have been invented to characterize modern man: the grave of desire that man digs for himself, or the grave which the desire digs for man, the grave of the voluptuaries.

"And Moses heard the people weeping, family by family, every man at the door of his tent; and the anger of the Lord was kindled greatly; and it was evil in Moses' eyes" (Num. 11:10). For the first time, Moses sees the people's actions as evil. He is no longer their defense attorney. This brought the great march to an end. The vision of the Messiah, of the Land of Israel, of redemption, became a distant one, like a star on a mysterious horizon. It twinkled, but the road suddenly became almost endless. Why does Moses now speak out of the depths of resignation and condemn the people? Why did he pray for them after the Golden Calf but not now?

The Pagan Lifestyle

The incident of Kivrot ha-Ta'avah differed greatly from that of the Golden Calf. The making of the calf was the result of great primitive fright. The people thought that Moses was dead; they were afraid of the desert and did not know what the future held in store for them. Overwhelmed by loneliness and terror, they violated the precept of *avodah zarah*, idolatry. There were mitigating circumstances: they wanted the Golden Calf to substitute for Moses, as the *Rishonim* say.

At Kivrot ha-Ta'avah, we encounter idolatry in a different sense. We must distinguish between *avodah zarah* as a ceremony or ritual and as a pagan way. Paganism is not only the worship of an idol; it encompasses more—a certain lifestyle. The pagan cries out for variety, for boundlessness, for unlimited lust and insatiable desire, for the demonic dream of total conquest, of drinking the cup of pleasure to its dregs. The pagan way of life is the very antithesis of Judaism, which demands limiting our enjoyment and, if necessary, stepping backward to withdraw and retreat. When people reach out for the unreachable, for the orgiastic and hypnotic, they do not violate the prohibition of *avodah zarah*, but they adopt the pagan way of life—and the Torah hates the pagan way of life more than it hates the idol.

The Torah describes beautifully the way in which the pagan gathers the quail to gratify his hungry senses:

> And the people rose up all that day, and all the night, and all the next day, and gathered the quails; he that gathered least gathered ten heaps; and they spread them out for themselves all around the camp (Num. 11:32).

They were mad with desire; nothing could control their desire for vastness. Their imagination excited them; their good sense was surrounded with a nimbus that was irresistible. The Jew eats in a measured way, only as much as is required, as with the manna; the pagan is impatient and insatiable. That is what the Torah describes in Kivrot ha-Ta'avah.

Moses' Intuition

With this, the triumphal final march suddenly came to a stop. The people who rejected the basic principle of limiting enjoyment were not worthy of entering the Land. Suddenly, the section of *Va-yehi bi-neso'a ha-aron* found itself dislocated. The distance to the land suddenly became very long. Of course, there was no edict yet concerning the forty years that the people would have to journey in the desert. But Moses felt intuitively that the great march had come to an end. His hopes would be unfulfilled, his visions unrealized, his prayers rejected.

I remember a similar experience during the illness of my wife. She was sick for four years. I am a realist, and it is very hard to fool me; but, somehow, I was convinced that somehow she would manage to get out of it, and I lived with hope and tremendous unlimited faith. However, the last Yom Kippur before she died, I was holding a *sefer Torah* for *Kol Nidrei*. When the *hazzan* finished *Kol Nidrei* and said the blessing *Sheheheyanu,* I turned over the *sefer Torah* to a student of mine and told him to put it in the *aron kodesh*. He put it in there, but apparently he did not place it well. The *sefer Torah* slipped and fell inside the *aron kodesh*. At that moment, I was filled with dreadful sense that nothing would help my wife's situation. And so it was.

When the people began to complain and to weep, Moses knew: This is the end; he will never see *Eretz Yisrael*, never! That is why he said: "If You will deal thus with me, kill me, I pray you, at once . . . and let me not look upon my wretchedness" (Num. 11:15). And how beautifully did our Rabbis interpret the verse: "And there ran a young man, and told Moses, and said: 'Eldad and Medad are prophesying in the camp'" (Num. 11:27). "And what were they saying? 'Moses will die and Joshua will lead the people into the Land'" (*Sifrei*, Num. 95).

It was then that *Vayehi bi-neso'a ha-aron* lost its place. Instead of the march bringing them closer to the Land of Israel, it took them away from the Promised Land. The *nun*s were inverted, and with the inversion Jewish history became inverted—and it is still inverted. The *parashah* is *still* dislocated. We cannot say "We are setting forth" with the same assurance and certitude that Moses displayed to his father-in-law—just twenty-four hours before the permissive multitude inverted the process of redemption. Due to this inversion, the messianic era did not commence in Moses' time, nor have we witnessed the fulfillment of the prophecy "On that day, the Lord will be one and His Name one" (Zech. 14:9).

❧ Miriam and the Spies

"Remember What God Did to Miriam"

A nd Miriam and Aaron spoke against Moses because
of the Cushite woman whom he had married. . . .
And they said: "Has the Lord indeed spoken only with
Moses? Has He not spoken also with us?" . . . And the
Lord spoke suddenly unto Moses, and unto Aaron, and
unto Miriam . . . and He said: "Hear now My words: if
there be a prophet among you, I the Lord do make Myself
known unto him in a vision, I do speak with him in a
dream. Not so My servant Moses; he is trusted in all My
house; with him do I speak mouth to mouth, even mani-
festly, and not in dark speeches; and the similitude of the
Lord does he behold; wherefore then were you not afraid
to speak against My servant, against Moses?" And the
anger of the Lord was kindled against them; and He
departed. And when the cloud was removed from over
the Tent, behold, Miriam was leprous, as white as snow
. . . (Num. 12: 1–10).

We are all familiar with Rashi's quotation from the *Midrash*

Tanhuma (*Shelah* 5) explaining why the story of the spies follows immediately the section dealing with Miriam's punishment: "Miriam was punished on account of the slander which she uttered against her brother; these sinners witnessed it, yet they did not learn a lesson from her" (Rashi, Num. 13:2, s.v. *shelah*). Indeed, the Torah tells us all, "Remember what God did to Miriam when you were on the way out of Egypt" (Deut. 24:9): remember and do not engage in slander.

Why did the Torah single out the sin of *lashon ha-ra*, evil speech or slander? In what respect does *lashon ha-ra* differ from other commandments concerning human relations, such as the prohibitions against perjury, stealing, taking revenge, or shaming somebody? And why did the Torah deem it necessary to include the incident of Miriam among the great events in Jewish history that we are commanded to remember, including the Exodus (Ex. 13:3), the Sabbath (Ex. 20:7), the revelation at Mount Sinai (Deut. 4:9–10), the Golden Calf (Deut. 9:7), and the war with Amalek (Deut. 25:17)?

"Miriam and Aaron spoke against Moses because of the Cushite woman whom he had married" (Num. 12:1). How shall we understand this? Miriam was the sister who, as a little girl, stood alone on the shore of the Nile to watch the floating ark. She had faith and hope even after her mother and father had resigned themselves and abandoned the baby. She and Aaron knew of Moses' greatness. How could they turn into accusers and prosecuting attorneys?

As *Hazal* tell us (*Sifrei*, Num. 99), the "Cushite woman" was Moses' wife Zipporah, who was unique and singular. Moses had separated from her because God had told him at Sinai, "You shall remain here with Me" (Deut. 5:28)—that is, withdraw from your family. Other people can go back to their jobs and to their homes, but Moses is different. Moses was elevated at Sinai to transcendental heights; he could not return to an earthly life. Miriam, however, considered Moses' separation from Zipporah to be unnecessary. Did not God speak with us as well, they asked. We were not told to separate from our spouses, so why was Moses told to do so?

Miriam and Aaron did not grasp the incommensurability of Moses' prophecy with that of other prophets. Moses spent forty days and nights on Sinai, where he did not eat or drink. He belonged to a different existential order of creation, one where the logos and ethos of other prophets do not apply. Their sin was in not understanding that he was the prophet *sui generis*, singular, unparalleled, and unmatched: "Not so My servant Moses" (Num. 12:7). Based on God's words to Miriam and Aaron, Maimonides codified the principle of the uniqueness of Mosaic prophecy both in *Hilkhot Yesodei ha-Torah* (7:6) and in his Thirteen Principles of Faith.

The Concept of Segullah

At this juncture, we come across a central idea in Judaism: *behirah*, chosenness or election. We believe that we are an *am ha-nivhar*, a chosen people. The Torah defines the concept of *behirah* by equating it with *segullah*: "You shall be a *segullah* to Me from among all the peoples" (Ex. 19:5). *Segullah* generally means treasure. I have many things, but there may be a certain thing that I treasure most amongst many treasures, one that I treat with special tenderness and care. The relation between me and this *segullah* is singular. There is an intrinsic, qualitative difference in the relationship. Jacob, of course, loved all his children, but Joseph was the *segullah*. There was a certain relationship between Joseph and Jacob that did not exist between Reuben and Jacob. It was not a question of intensity; it was rather a question of kind, of quality.

The *segullah* cannot be broken down into its component parts in order to be analyzed. The one who knew and recognized this was Judah. In his confrontation with Joseph (Gen. 44:18–34), Judah said, "His soul is bound up with the lad's soul" (Gen. 44:30). In other words, Jacob's love for Benjamin resulted in a metaphysical union of souls. Similarly, the Midrash explains that the verse, "These are the generations of Jacob: Joseph . . ." (Gen. 37:2), teaches that "The countenance of Joseph resembled Jacob, and everything that happened to Jacob happened to Joseph" (Gen. Rabbah 84:6). By hyphenating Jacob and Joseph, *Hazal* express their ontological unity; the I-awareness of Jacob included Joseph. His love for his other children, however deep and intense, did not precipitate oneness with them. Jacob's love for Rachel was special and unique, and he united metaphysically and ontologically only with her children, Joseph and Benjamin.

Aaron and Miriam, from the very outset, did not recognize the significance of the *segullah* element in Moses. They did not know that Moses merited special attention and deserved to be treated separately. That is why the Torah warns us not to compare Moses with other prophets.

We also understand now why the Torah, while reminding us of the Miriam episode, adds words that are *prima facie* unnecessary: "Remember what God did to Miriam *when you were on the way out of Egypt*" (Deut. 24:9). We all know the locus of the Exodus; why include this phrase? The Torah here tried to impress upon us that the whole Exodus never would have occurred had Moses not been a prophet and leader beyond the reach of the imagination. To liberate the people from Egypt, the leader had to speak on behalf of the Holy One. Only Moses could achieve that distinction; neither Aaron nor Miriam could. The *segullah* element in the Jewish people was responsible for the fulfillment of the promise that God made to Abraham, and the *segullah* element in Moses made it possible for an individual to represent the Almighty in acting to redeem the people. Remember, says the Torah, you are marching to the Promised Land as you leave Egypt. You were taken out of the land of Egypt because you had a *segullah* potential, and because the leader who took you out, who represents God, possesses the *segullah* quality. Miriam denied it, and you must remember not to deny it.

Motherly Devotion

There is an additional element to Moses' uniqueness. Moses knew well that God had not elected him as a diplomat, as a negotiator, but as the teacher or *rebbi* of the people, their spiritual and moral leader. However, until the incident at Kivrot ha-Ta'avah, which occurred shortly before Miriam's slander, he did not expect that he would assume the role of an *omen*, a nursing parent (Num. 11:12). The teacher does instruct his disciple, but the disciple very seldom becomes a part of him. When the mother teaches the baby, the baby becomes a part of her. When she rears the baby, the mother has but one calling, one purpose: to protect the baby. The *omen* forgoes personal life; the *omen* belongs to the infant.

Moses discovered that teaching is not enough for a leader of Israel. His job is nursing, carrying the baby in his arms, watching every step, guessing the baby's needs, feeling pain when the baby cries and being happy when the baby is cheerful. Moses, who was reconciled with his role as a teacher and leader of adults, began to doubt his ability to play the role of an *omen*. It entailed the tragic realization that from now on he had no rights at all. He was not entitled to enjoy life as an individual, to be happy in an ordinary way, like any other human being. This is why *Hazal* tell us that "he separated from his wife." He lost his family; he became the mother-nurse of the Jewish people with no family of his own. There was a census taken in the desert at the beginning and again at the end of the forty years. Moses' children are not mentioned once. He no longer had children of his own; he was the *omen* of the entire community.

Moses realized this during the incident at Kivrot ha-Ta'avah. And that is what Miriam, the true, loyal sister, resented. Does prophecy require of man alienation from his family, she asked. Does God require of the prophet that he forget his sister and brother, his children and wife, and dedicate himself only to the people? "Has He not spoken also with us"—and we live a beautiful life with our spouses and children and relatives. It does not interfere with our devotion to the people.

The Almighty meted out her punishment with strictness and speed. He told her: There is a difference between you and Moses. An ordinary prophet does not have to sacrifice his private interests, his selfish concerns, his family, his father, mother, children, brother, sister; he can be a prophet, communicate with God, and at the same time be a devoted father, a loving brother, and a helpful head of the family. "Not so My servant Moses." He is consecrated fully and wholly to Me.

The Spies' Mission

Now let us pick up the sin of the *meraggelim*, the spies. The whole episode is puzzling. First, why was it necessary to send the spies at all? What were they supposed to do? What kind of report did Moses expect from them? The report they brought was the truth. Why, then, were they severely punished? We understand the horrible sin of the Golden Calf, but what was the sin of the spies?

As a matter of fact, their mission was not to spy, *leraggel*, but rather "*latur et ha-aretz*, to scout the land" (Num. 13:16). The difference between *leraggel* and *latur* is quite obvious. *Leraggel* means spying to find out the military weak spots in the defense system of a potential enemy. Joseph accuses his brothers of being spies: "*Meraggelim attem*, You are spies, you came to see the nakedness of the land" (Gen. 42:9). Nothing of that sort was entrusted to the twelve scouts. Their assignment, spelled out by Moses, was to search and explore, to scout. It was not military intelligence but a study mission. They were to see the land (Num. 13:18), and after their return they were to submit a number of reports. One was a demographic report: Are the people strong or weak, few or many (ibid.)? The other was an agricultural study: Is the soil rich or poor (13:20)? Moses needed no military intelligence when the Jews left Egypt, and he needed none here. Moses knew very well that the entry to the Land of Israel would be accompanied by miracles, as was the Exodus. There was no need to send them to collect intelligence data. Why did he send them to study the land and the people?

In my opinion, Moses acted in accordance with the principle that one must not propose to, let alone wed, a woman he does not know, no matter how highly recommended (*Kiddushin* 41a). The Bible tells us, "And the servant told Isaac all the things that he had done. And Isaac brought her into his mother Sarah's tent, and took Rebecca, and she became his wife" (Gen. 24:66–67). Notwithstanding the servant's portrayal of Rebecca's wisdom, intelligence, hospitality, and kindness, Isaac did not take her for a wife immediately. As Rashi interprets the verses (24:67, s.v. *ha-ohelah*), Isaac brought her into Sarah's tent before marrying her in order to see if she was a worthy successor to Sarah. Would she restore the glory and the pristine beauty of Sarah's tent? Isaac waited to see if the same cloud would return to the tent, if the yeast in the dough would rise, if the candle would be relit. When Isaac saw that all had returned, he married Rebecca. Eliezer was trustworthy, devoted, and loyal, but still, Isaac did not wed Rebecca until he became convinced that she was the equal of Sarah.

Marriage is not an ordinary transaction. It is not just a civil commitment or a mundane partnership. It is an existential commitment, a covenantal union. Two lonely people join their souls. Two strangers decide to unite their destinies, to share the same fate, to suffer and rejoice together, to travel together and pay the toll of the road jointly. When one takes on such an all-inclusive, all-encompassing commitment, one cannot trust anybody, no matter how loyal and trustworthy the other person might be.

The Jews at this time were ready to march to the Promised Land. The entry into the Land of Israel, we have to understand, was not just a physical act of crossing the Jordan River. It was a marriage between a people and a land, a union of the rocky hills and the sandy trails with a people returning to its origin.

The entry signified the destiny of a people united with the destiny of a land. Consequently, the people could not just enter the land without meeting it first. They knew it was a land of milk and honey, but they had to experience it and get acquainted with it before they became united. That is why, a short time before the planned entry into the Promised Land, Moses sent explorers to study the land—not to gather intelligence data, which was completely unnecessary. He sent the would-be groom to meet and to see the would-be bride.

Out of the Valley of Hebron

Moses tells the explorers to "Go up here into the Negev, and go up into the mountains" (Num. 13:17). In telling them how to travel, Moses revealed to the explorers the reason why he was sending them and of what their mission consisted. But in order to understand this, we must turn back to the story of Joseph's being sent by Jacob to inquire about the welfare of his brothers in Shechem. "Jacob sent Joseph *me-emek Hevron*, out of the valley of Hebron, and he came to Shechem" (Gen. 37:14). Rashi comments (s.v. *me-emek*),

> But was not Hebron situated on a hill, as it is said (Num. 13:22), "And they went up from the Negev and reached Hebron"? Rather, [the meaning is that Jacob sent him] in consequence of the [necessity of bringing into operation the] profound (*amukah*) thought of the righteous man who was buried in Hebron—in order that there might be fulfilled that which was spoken to Abraham [when the covenant was made] "between the parts."

The Midrash saw in the words *"emek Hevron"* great symbolism. One who finds himself in a valley over which tall mountains tower can see very little. He lives in shadow; his field of vision is very limited. However, a person standing on the peak of the mountain can encompass with his glance a very large area. His field of vision is enormous. Standing on the plateau, on the peak of the mountain, he can observe things he could not see while he was in the valley. When one climbs up to the top of a tall mountain, one suddenly sees new horizons, new scenery and landscapes, charming and attractive.

Jacob did not just send Joseph; he accompanied him for part of the road and then down the slope into the depression of Hebron. Jacob was completely unaware of the consequences this errand would produce. He was in a valley, he did not see far enough. His intuition, his outlook, his glance, usually embraced enormous areas, but not this time, not on that day. Had Jacob had his incisive intuition, he would never have sent Joseph at all. Jacob knew very well that Joseph was disliked; to send Joseph to Shechem to inquire about the health and welfare of his brothers was foolhardy. But Jacob was in a valley, *emek Hevron*. Had he been on the peak of the mountain as he usually was, had he been inspired that day, he would never have lost Joseph. But he descended with Joseph from the peak of the mountain into the valley, into the depression, and his view became obscured. He sent Joseph, and in sending Joseph he also precipitated the exile in Egypt.

The history of Jewish exile started the very moment Jacob turned his back on Joseph. And now, Moses said, we are elected to carry out another assignment, a much more pleasant and joyful one. We are elected to climb up the mount, to stop on its peak and cast a searching glance. We belong not to the waiting generations, but to the fulfilling generation. That is what Moses said to the twelve would-be explorers: Jacob came down the mount, you go up the mount. You will see something which Jacob did not see. You will see that the people are returning to the land.

Moses told them, "Go up . . . the Negev." The Negev is the cradle of Jewish history. The "covenant between the pieces" most probably took place in the Negev. The Negev pulled Abraham, "*halokh ve-nasoa ha-negbah*, going on still toward the

Negev" (Gen. 12:9). This is the spot where the great covenant was concluded between God, man, and land. Now, said Moses, go and reverse Jacob's movement. Go not from the peak of the mount into the depression, but from the valley unto the peak of the mount. And when you stand at the peak of the mount, *"u-re'item et ha-aretz mah hi,* and see the land, what it is" (Num. 13:18). This was not a question but a prediction: you will see what the land is. You will encounter a great vision, a wondrous spectacle. You will realize the link between God and the land, and understand that there is perfect harmony and an eternal bond. You will understand the quality and the essence of the land that is the abode of the *Shekhinah,* that only there can the people realize their great potential. You will see that the land is worthy of our sacrifices, our waiting, our faith, our hope. The uniqueness and singularity of *Eretz Yisrael* can somehow be united with the element of *segullah*, the uniqueness and singularity of the people.

"They went up from the Negev and reached Hebron" (Num. 13:22). Eleven explorers did not care even to enter Hebron. They did not go up the mount from which Jacob descended into the valley. They did not get a comprehensive view of the land. There was no revelation of its exalted grandeur and glory. They just explored it in a piecemeal fashion, "from the wilderness of Zin unto Rehob, at the entrance to Hamath" (Num. 13:21). They did not understand the *segullah* charisma of the land and of the people. They never reported back to Moses concerning their mission, *"U-re'item et ha-aretz ma hi,"* to see what was unique about the land. Only Caleb and Joshua reported that "The land is very good" (Num. 14:7). She is worthy. It behooves us to wed the land, to be united in an indissoluble union. We have no other land, for our destiny is linked up with the destiny of the land.

Overlooking Segullah

This is exactly what the *Midrash Tanhuma*, quoted by Rashi (Num. 13:2), meant when it said that the spies should have taken a lesson from Miriam. It was not the lesson of *lashon ha-ra*, of not engaging in slander. Miriam had overlooked the *segullah* element in Moses, and they overlooked the *segullah* element in the land. Miriam ignored the chosenness of her brother Moses, his numinous character and charisma. The spies, likewise, could not grasp the secret of a *segullah* land and its unique metaphysical relationship to the people. There was a common denominator in the two episodes, in her protest against Moses and in their report submitted to Moses. The element of *segullah* was absent from both.

Segullah is to be found in the Creator Himself. Maimonides repeats many times (e.g., *Hilkhot Yesodei ha-Torah* 1:1–7) that the Almighty is not only one, but He is the only one, the single one. On the one hand, God is the origin of everything. Wherever one finds being, one finds the Almighty. *Ehyeh Asher Ehyeh* (Ex. 3:14)—wherever there is existence, the Almighty is present. To exist means to be in the heart of eternity. Whoever is hugged and embraced by eternity, by the Almighty, exists. There is unity between creation and Creator.

On the other hand, God is alone, different in the ultimate sense of the word from the world. God not only sustains the world, He also negates the world and all being. If there is being, it is only the true Being of the Almighty. No one can imitate the Holy One or say that he shares in divine Being, since divine Being is exclusive. From the perspective of the Holy One, the world does not exist.

Since man was created in the image of God, man too has a dialectical existence. He is a part of the universal order but is, as well, a single *segullah* individual. We may compare man with other creatures, with the brute in the field and the tree in the forest. But at the same time man remains an outsider, a stranger who has nothing in common with nature. Within society, there is a dual role in the relationship between man and man. On the one hand, man is told by the Torah to practice *hesed*, to tear down the barriers surrounding the egocentric individual, to let others enter his private lodging and share everything with them. What is *hesed* if not an open existence—Abraham sat with his tent open to all (Gen. 18:1). On the other hand, man is also urged by the Torah to guard his uniqueness and his singular endowment. Man, according to Judaism, is supposed to live in two domains, public and private, *reshut ha-rabbim* and *reshut ha-yahid*. If man lives only in his private domain, he becomes an egotist. If he lives only in the public domain, he loses his *segullah* element and becomes an imitator and nothing else. He loses his originality and inspiration.

Moses was the great leader who was one of the crowd. He suffered for the many. The capacity to suffer for others—as he did for Miriam—is the first prerequisite of the leader. Faced with the sin of the Golden Calf, Moses asked God to erase his name from God's book (Ex. 32:32). He was willing to sacrifice his life, his very existence, for his people. He lived an open and dutiful life, all-encompassing, all-loving. He did not display his *segullah* when he dealt with simple people. "And it came to pass on the morrow, that Moses sat to judge the people; and the people stood about Moses from the morning to the evening" (Ex. 18:13). He personified all the dreams, all the hopes, all the desires of the people. He suffered with them; he rejoiced with them.

However, there was also a *segullah* element in Moses. He was lonely, and at times he could not communicate with others. He led a *segullah* existence, one inimitable, unmatched, practically incomprehensible to others. "Now Moses would take the tent and pitch it outside the camp" (Ex. 33:7). When Moses was in the public domain, he merged with the people; and when he was in the private domain, he was alone with the Creator. This mode of existence finds its complete harmony in the Holy One, but as far as human beings are concerned, we are dialectical beings.

We cannot understand the ends which revolve about *segullah*. There is an element of the numinous, of the frighteningly strange, of the hidden and ineffable, in the *segullah* charisma.

Why did the Holy One choose us as a *segullah* nation? Why was *Eretz Yisrael* selected as the land of the *segullah* nation and itself endowed with the *segullah* quality? This remains an enigma. We fail to grasp why a *segullah* nation is supposed to live hundreds of years in exile. When values are comparable, when common denominators unite many values, the mind is capable of understanding. However, *segullah* is beyond and above the capacity of the logos to comprehend. At certain times, when the *segullah* element is in the background, history is simple and understandable. At other times, there is revelation of the *segullah* element. At such a moment, the enigma rises and everything becomes mysterious. The *segullah* element cannot be understood; it can only be lived and experienced through an act of faith. It cannot be conceived through an intellectual gesture.

With regard to the mitzvah of *tzitzit*, we are told: "Put upon the fringe of each corner a thread of *tekhelet*, and it shall be for you a fringe that you may look upon and remember" (Num. 15:38–39). *Tekhelet* and *lavan,* blue and white, represent two approaches of man to himself and to the world outside himself. *Lavan* in classical Hebrew signifies white as a color, but it also signifies clarity, distinctiveness, and openness. It denotes rationality, simplicity, and truthfulness, something which is obvious to everybody as an elementary truth. *Tekhelet* is just the opposite. *Hazal* said: "*Tekhelet* resembles the sea, and the sea resembles the sky, and the sky resembles the celestial throne" (*Sotah* 17a). They were associating blue with distance and inapproachability. The blue sky is very distant; the blue sea is wide and endless. And, of course, the throne of God is beyond the universe. Whatever we cannot reach, whatever is outside our control, whatever suggests mystery to us, is considered by *Hazal* as *tekhelet*.

A Jew is expected to focus his glance on the white and attempt to understand the world. The Torah does not want people to live in obscurity. It encourages man to explore all the phenomena of nature, to use his mind and make discoveries, to be scientifically oriented and technologically minded.

On the other hand, one thread in the *tzitzit* is blue. Man sometimes meets with mystery, with something numinous and awesome, something beyond the bounds of the rational and intelligible. We encounter unexpectedly the *segullah* quality; everything becomes distant and strange, remote as the sky and distant from our minds. But we have been trained to accept both. If the experience is understandable, then our intellect interprets the experience. If the experience is not understandable, unintelligible, we interpret it through an act of faith, "That you may look upon it, and remember all the commandments of the Lord" (Num. 15:39).

❧ The Korah Rebellion

The Character of the Controversy

The Korah rebellion was a unique event. Prior to it, the people complained, protested, and murmured—but always in response to a physical need, a biological pressure (such as hunger or thirst), a primitive fear of an enemy or fiend, be it Amalek, a serpent, or simply the wilderness itself. Primitive man is afraid not only of human beings, but of anything unannounced. "The children of Israel lifted their eyes, and, behold, the Egyptians were marching after them; and they were greatly frightened, and the children of Israel cried unto the Lord" (Ex. 14:10). Fear prompted their cry of protest. "When they came to Marah they could not drink the waters of Marah, for they were bitter . . . and the people murmured against Moses" (Ex. 15:23–24). Thirst prompted their protest. "The whole congregation of the children of Israel murmured against Moses and Aaron . . . 'Would we had died by the hand of the Lord in the land of Egypt, when we sat by the fleshpots and when we did eat bread to satisfaction'" (Ex. 16:2–3). They were hungry, and hungry people are angry and strident. "The congregation journeyed . . . and encamped in Rephidim, and there was no water for the people to drink; and the people quarreled with Moses, and said, 'Give us water that we may drink'" (Ex. 17:1–2).

There were no political disagreements with Moses, no ideological controversies, no rebellions. There were only protests, complaints, and quarrels. All these were consequences of the discomfort and hardship to which they were subjected during the first and second years that they sojourned in the desert. They wanted water and food; they were afraid and they protested. Even the Golden Calf episode was not precipitated by idolatrous ideas that corroded the moral fiber of the people and influenced their philosophy. The Golden Calf, rather, was precipitated by the primitive, instinctual horror that befalls a lost sheep in wide open spaces. It was a spontaneous reaction to the primordial terror of being lost, leaderless, in the wilderness. They thought that Moses would never return, and without Moses how could they survive? "And they said to [Aaron], 'Arise, make us gods that will go before us, for this man Moses who took us out of the land of Egypt, we know not what is become of him' " (Ex. 32:1).

In a word, all the previous quarrels were unorganized, unplanned, spontaneous reactions to situations they confronted and did not know how to handle. The quarrels were generated by a mob mentality, which easily gets excited but also easily regains its equilibrium.

The Korah controversy was of a totally different character. It was a rebellion, not a quarrel due to ungratified physical desires. Moreover, the masses were not involved at all. The *am*, the people, that demanded water at Rephidim, the *am* that told Aaron to build a God, did not participate in the anti-Moses campaign of Korah. The leadership of the rebellion consisted of a few individuals, and the followers were several hundred at most. These people were of the elite, the aristocracy, "princes of the congregation, elect men of the assembly, men of renown" (Num. 16:2). It was a conspiracy, premeditated and carefully thought out. In understanding the history and motivation of this rebellion, I believe we should follow Nahmanides.

Nahmanides explains that Korah's enmity was incurred when Aaron was elevated to the position of high priest. However, in spite of his anger, Korah did not attempt to come out publicly against Moses. He understood very well that the people, notwithstanding minor incidents, were devoted and loyal to their great leader, and that any attempt to unseat Moses would be met with anger and derision. Korah waited patiently for an opportunity that would somehow undermine Moses' position and popularity.

Korah Seizes an Opportunity

The opportune moment arrived sooner than Korah anticipated. It was the incident of the spies, perhaps the most tragic incident in Moses' life. The Almighty's decree that all the adults would die in the desert was a hard blow to Moses' prestige. For a short while, he lost his influence over the crowds. Before the Children of Israel had left Egypt, while they were still busy building fortresses for Pharaoh, Moses had promised those slaves that a short time after their departure from Egypt they would enter into the Promised Land, a land flowing with milk and honey. Indeed, they were ready to invade the Negev the second year after the Exodus. Suddenly all their hopes and dreams were dissipated and shattered. No land, no conquest, no rivers of milk and honey, no realizations of the promise were in sight—only many bleak and dreary years before Israel would set foot on the soil of Canaan.

Where is Moses' pledge, the people asked each other; where is his clairvoyance, his prescience, his prophecy? When Moses invited Dathan and Abiram to come over, they said, "You have not brought us into a land flowing with milk and honey, nor have you given us an inheritance of fields and vineyards" (Num. 16:14). Moses, your promise has not come true. Moses' popularity was at a low ebb. The time has arrived, said Korah, to act. Korah started to recruit disgruntled and frustrated people, organizing a formidable opposition to Moses.

Rashi offers two interpretations of the opening phrase "*Va-yikkah Korah*"—literally, "Korah took" (Num. 16:1, s.v. *va-yikkah*). The first is: "He betook himself on one side with the intention of separating himself from the community so that he might raise a protest regarding the priesthood." Then Korah made the final leap. Until then, no one had dared to impugn Moses' authority. Korah was the first to separate himself from a community which was committed to Moses and revered him. Rashi's phrase "*lakah et atzmo*" also indicates that Korah dedicated himself completely to that task. There was only one goal in Korah's life: to unseat Moses. He dedicated his whole self to this diabolical plan of undermining Moses' exalted position within the community.

Rashi's second interpretation is that Korah took others with him. In the beginning he did not reveal anything to his prospective co-conspirators. But when the divine decree condemning the Jews to the forty-year sojourn in the wilderness was announced, he thought that a golden opportunity had presented itself and he revealed his plans to Dathan, Abiram, and others. Rashi's second interpretation was that "he attracted the heads of the courts with words," by using clever and intelligent words. He began to conspire, to criticize Moses, to attack and ridicule. He used all the weapons in his arsenal. In conversation with some, he was serious; in conversation with others, he was humorous. With some, he played the role of persecutor; with others, the role of champion of justice.

Rashi says (s.v. *ve-Datan*) that the tribe of Reuben became involved because they lived next door to Korah. "*Oy le-rasha, oy li-shekeno.*" They met Korah too often, and he succeeded in convincing them. Nahmanides (s.v. *va-yikah*) mentions that Korah appealed to the tribe of the firstborn, who bore a grudge against Moses because they felt that the privileges of the priesthood belonged to them.

However, any conspiracy or organized rebellion, no matter how egotistically motivated, must develop an ideology in order to succeed. Korah planned an anti-Moses movement, and such a movement cannot exist or make headway without developing an ideology. Every movement must have a motto, and Korah indeed provided the philosophy of the rebellion.

Individual and Communal Holiness

Korah's first argument, which the Torah states at the very beginning of the story, was, "You have gone too far, for all the community is holy, and the Lord is in their midst; why then do you raise yourself above the congregation of the Lord?" (Num. 16:3). The basis of this challenge was very simple and, at first glance, quite logical. No one can deny Korah's assertion that the whole community is holy; it is the very essence of our chosenness. Every Jew possesses intrinsic sanctity. As far as holiness is concerned, there is no distinction between Moses and a simple woodchopper. Hence, Korah asked, what right did Moses or Aaron have to lead, to guide, to rule? He charged them with seizing power illegitimately. He raised the millennia-old argument based on the equality of all people.

Korah was wrong. He was unaware of the twofold character of *kedushat Yisrael*, the sanctity of Israel, and of the mystery of the dual *kedushah*. Note Rashi's comment (s.v. *ki*) to "You are a holy nation, *am kadosh*, to the Lord your God; and the Lord has chosen you to be a cherished people, *am segullah*, unto Himself" (Deut. 14:2). Rashi apparently questioned the duplication in the verse, and he explained, " 'You are a holy nation'—your holiness comes to you from your fathers. In addition [to that sanctity], 'The Lord has chosen you [to be a cherished people unto Himself].' " In other words, there is the twofold idea of *kedushat Yisrael*.

First, the community as a whole is holy. *Kenesset Yisrael* is not just a conglomerate of people, not just a multitude of souls; it is an individuality, an entity unto itself, a personality. The sanctity of our covenantal community is inherited from our ancestors. In order to lay claim to sanctity, the individual must draw upon the resources of sanctity available to the community. If the individual derives his sanctity from the community, then Moses derived as much sanctity from the community as did the simple woodchopper. From this perspective, every Jew's sanctity would be commensurate and equal. This sanctity is not personal and intimate, but is a universal, community-rooted, and community-nourished holiness inherited from one's progenitors.

However, Judaism was not satisfied with the social aspect of *kedushah*. If the community were the only source of sanctity, then the individual would be deprived of his creative role, his individual initiative, his originality and uniqueness. The outstanding person would not be able to develop into a great leader. Hence, the Torah says, there is a second resource of *kedushah*— the sanctity which the individual detects in the inner recesses of his personality. No one else has a sanctity like his; an individual's sanctity cannot be shared with somebody else. To paraphrase *Hazal* (*Berakhot* 58a), just as people have different ideas, so they have different *kedushot*. There is a separate *kedushah* attached to every individual.

From this viewpoint, the community derives *kedushah* by integrating the countless *kedushah* experiences of the individual members of the community. The single person sanctifies the community.

How beautifully, then, did the Torah state, "For you are a holy nation to the Lord your God" (Deut. 14:2): you are holy because you are a member of a holy nation. "*Am kadosh atah*": the nation precedes the individual in this part of the verse. But at the same time, "*u-vekha bahar Hashem lihyot lo le-am segullah*" (ibid.): *u-vekha*, you the individual, *bahar Hashem*, God has charged, *lihyot*, to form or create, *lo le-am segullah*, a treasured people unto Him. In the second part of the verse, the individual—*u-vekha*—precedes the nation—*am segullah*; God has charged every individual with the mission to create a treasured people.

It is obvious that as far as the election of individuals is concerned, their endowments cannot be equal. Each individual receives the endowment which reflects the greatness of his or her personality. The individual *kedushah* experiences are incommensurate with each other; they are proportional to the individual's involvement and dedication, as well as to the individual's depth and sweep. This *kedushah* is an expression of one's greatness, and not all people are alike as far as greatness is concerned.

The statement by Korah that "All the community is holy" is correct as long as we are speaking of the community-rooted *kedushah* inherited from our ancestors. Indeed, "all the community," the community as a whole, is a source of holiness. Moses was born into a Jewish community as was the baby of a slave. Their shares in the endowment of sanctity were equal. However, if we shift our attention from the social aspect to the individual aspect of *kedushah*, the whole idea of equality turns into an absurdity. We must admit that the *behirah* of Moses was above and beyond the *behirah* of the woodchopper or water-drawer.

Interesting is the response Moses gave Korah: "Come morning (*boker*), the Lord will make known who is His and who is holy, and will grant him access to Himself; He will grant access to the one He has chosen" (Num. 16:5). Moses speaks not of the congregation, but of an individual. As far as personalistic *behirah* is concerned, there is a difference between individual and individual. Medieval grammarians such as Radak (*Sefer ha-Shorashim*, s.v. *bkr*) pointed out that *boker* has the connotation of discriminating and differentiating between individual forms. *Boker* means the period of recognition of things, events, and people. *Erev*, evening, in contradistinction, is the time of monotony and uniformity. *Erev* is a time of apprehending the surroundings as one amorphous, formless mass where individuals merge into one homogeneous, black reality.

Moses said to Korah, Your concept of *kedushah* is identical with the *erev*, with the bleakness of an eternal night whose darkness and dreariness envelop everything. All you see is one piece of formless reality called *edah*, community. You do not see individuals. Your concept of *kedushah* is limited to what the medieval philosophers call *homer ha-hiyuli*, the primordial mixture. From the viewpoint of *erev*, your argument is valid. However, there is another idea of the holy, the personal, individualistic holiness in which the human personality participates with all its singular greatness and beauty. This is the holiness which discriminates, which sees individuals. This is the holiness of the morning, *boker*, when the world emerges from the nightly anonymity into a world full of sun, joy, individual freedom, and individual greatness. As far as this holiness is concerned, the crowd is far below the individual, and each person is consecrated to a unique task that only he can perform.

Conversion, with its two basic acts of circumcision and immersion in a *mikveh,* symbolically represents the two dimensions of *kedushah*—the universal, community-rooted concept and the individual one. Through circumcision the convert becomes integrated into the community, and by doing so he is given the opportunity to draw upon the communal social resources of *kedushah* and to be a component part of the community. Immersion is indicative of personal commitment. It is associated with *kabbalat ol mitzvot*, taking on a personal commitment to God's commandments. The convert separates himself from the community for a short time. He retreats into isolation, hiding in the waters, and accepts responsibility as an individual and not as a member of the community.

The Political and Teaching Communities

Korah charged that Moses and Aaron were power-hungry, that they had set up a power structure and raised themselves above the congregation. He equated the exercise of power with kingship. This equation and the politicization of the relationship between the leader and those whom he leads is incorrect. The covenantal community is, first and foremost, not a political community; it is a teaching community. Throughout the ages, the central figure in the covenantal community has not been a king, warrior, or high priest, but the teacher, the *rebbi*. The people are not subjects, as is customary in the political community; they are disciples. The relationship is not of a political nature, nor is it connected to the use of violence or the employment of sanctions. It is a free commitment on the part of the disciples to their master and teacher. The latter does not impose any authority upon the disciples. No one asks them to obey his words and to follow him. They can terminate the relationship at any time.

Basically, Judaism disapproves of all forms of human government. There are definite streaks of political anarchism in our reluctance to recognize man as king. God governs; no one else may usurp this prerogative. The only power structure that Judaism has accepted is the non-institutionalized relationship prevailing between teacher and student. Moses is not known to us as a monarch, even though he was formally a king—"When there was a king in Jeshurun" (Deut. 33:5). He was known as *Mosheh Rabbenu*, as the greatest of all teachers, the teacher par excellence. Aaron is not just a high priest; he, too, is a great teacher. The priests themselves are not just charismatic personalities; their sanctity is associated with teaching: "They shall teach Your ordinances to Jacob, and Your law to Israel" (Deut. 33:10); "For the priest's lips shall keep knowledge, and they will seek the law at his mouth" (Mal. 2:7). The disciples love their masters and listen, not to their orders, since they give none, but to their teachings, which enlighten the mind and gladden the heart. Moses had not raised himself above the community, as Korah charged, but the community raised him above itself. Moses was elevated without questing for leadership. The teacher is certainly elected by God to be near Him, and his personal *kedushah* transcends that of his disciples. A saintly person is the leader because he is the teacher.

The Autonomy of Halakhic Thought

Now let us pick up Korah's second argument. The second argument of Korah is not mentioned in the Bible. Rashi (Num. 16:1, s.v. *ve-Datan*) quotes from *Tanhuma* (*Korah* 2) and tells the following story: Korah attired two hundred and fifty chiefs of the court in robes of *tekhelet*, purple-blue. They stood before Moses and said to him: "Is a garment that is entirely of *tekhelet* subject to the law of *tzitzit*, or is it exempt?" Moses answered, "It is subject to the law," whereupon they began to jeer at him: "Is that possible? In a robe of any different-colored material, one thread of *tekhelet* exempts it; should not the robe that is entirely of *tekhelet* be exempt?"

The Midrash (*Tanhuma*, loc. cit.) tells us another story, which is similar to the first. Korah asked, "Must one attach a *mezuzah* to the doorpost of a house filled with Torah scrolls?" Moses answered in the affirmative. They jeered again and said: "Is it possible that two short sections—*Shema* and *Ve-haya im shamoa*—are enough for a house, while a multitude of Torah scrolls does not suffice?"

These two stories have a common motif. The Midrash, using sarcasm and humor, exposes the whole philosophy of Korah and his goals. All Jews are equal, he said; hence, everyone is entitled to interpret the law. Korah wanted not only political power—he wanted to succeed Moses as *rebbi*, so that countless generations afterwards should say *Korah rabbenu*. He impugned and challenged not only Moses' political authority, but his halakhic authority as well. The study of the law and its interpretation, Korah argued, are exoteric, democratic acts, in which every intelligent person may engage. Moses' claim to be the exclusive legal authority and exclusive interpreter of the law, Korah argued, was unfounded and unwarranted.

The consequence of such a "democratic" philosophy is obvious. What Korah wanted—and what many want even now, whether they state it clearly or use equivocal terms and dubious language to cover it up—is for the instrument of interpretation of the Torah to be common sense, the everyday empirical intelligence, and not the esoteric, conceptualizing logos which can be attained only through painstaking study and hard training. Korah argued that every Jew with common sense should have the right to interpret the laws of the Torah and determine halakhic matters in commonsense categories.

Under the aspect of common sense, Korah's argument against Moses' decision was valid. If one purple thread is sufficient, why should a purple garment require *tzitzit*? If one can fulfill the mitzvah of *mezuzah* by attaching two *parashiyyot* to the door, why should not the presence of many scrolls in a house exempt the latter from the need of a *mezuzah*?

However, *Torah she-be-al peh*, the Oral Law, cannot be identified with common sense. It has a methodology of its own; it has a singular approach, a distinct form of analysis, its own categories, and its own strange schemata. Can common sense explain that a king is disqualified as a formal witness? Are Moses, King David, King Solomon, and the King Messiah all inferior to a simple Sabbath-observant woodchopper? Is there a commonsense reason to exclude women from being formal witnesses, when the Bible itself tells us that man and woman were both created in the image of God and takes for granted their equality? However, the *Torah she-be-al peh* has its own methods of conceptualization. The halakhist works, like the mathematician, in an *a priori* world. His constructs are ideal. He does not merely study reality; he prepares abstract schemata and applies them to the world of sense.

Aristotelian physics, which unfortunately dominated Western thought throughout antiquity and in the Middle Ages, failed miserably because its foundation was common sense. The great accomplishment of Galileo and Newton consisted in replacing the practical, commonsense approach with the conceptualizing, creative scientific logos. The scientific logos conceptualizes reality; the commonsense logos takes reality at face value. Galileo and Newton proclaimed the principle of mathematization and quantification of reality, of converting sense qualities like heat, light, color, and sound into quantitative mathematical relations. Aristotle, for instance, said that all things fall downwards because they are heavy. In other words, he considered the gravitational pull a result of heaviness or weight. This is nonsense; the reverse is true: weight is the consequence of the gravitational pull. Newton discarded common sense and approached the matter from the viewpoint of the esoteric, abstract, creative conceptualizing logos, and he came up with his famous formula, $F = G(m_1)(m_2)/r^2$. In other words, gravitational pull is nothing but a mathematical relation between two bodies, which consists of the product of the masses over the square of the distance. This method of quantification was perhaps the greatest discovery in the annals of mankind. Had mankind remained satisfied with Aristotelian physics, we could not have gone to the moon.

Mathematics is not just a corpus of equations, nor is physics merely a collection of natural laws; mathematics and physics are methods of thinking, a unique logos. So too is the *Torah she-be-al peh*. It is not merely a compilation of laws. Of course, its laws and statutes are of utmost significance. However, if we discard the view that *Torah she-be-al peh* is a system of thought structures and unique logical categories which are accessible to the human mind only if the latter is ready to subject itself to rigid training, we open up the floodgates and any ignoramus may claim authority, as did Korah.

Act and Experience

The adherents of "commonsense Halakhah" are misled by a basic philosophical doctrine. They expound a theory of religious subjectivism. *Prima facie*, it is hard to refute this theory, because it contains a kernel of truth. God, this theory says, is interested in the heart, in man's inner world. Faith, fundamentally, is an inner experience. Man meets God in the mysterious recesses of his personality. The God-experience is iridescent, dynamic, bold; it breaks out to the exterior of the human personality and turns into an objective deed, into action.

In a word, this theory claims that the *mitzvot* manifest an inner mood, a spiritual quest. The *mitzvot*, it claims, are supposed to reflect the inner experience; they are external correlates which run parallel to the experiential order. If this theory is correct, its adherents argue, then the *mitzvot* must correspond in the most consonant way to the mood they are supposed to express. Hence, the *mitzvot* must avail themselves of the media of expression which are best fitted to reflect the inner experience. And, they argue, scholars who live in a world of abstractions cannot determine the redemptive power of *mitzvot*; only a commonsense approach is capable of gauging the therapeutic energy of each mitzvah and utilizing it in the most efficient manner.

Korah said to Moses: The *tekhelet* thread was meant as a reminder of the mysterious link between the blue sea and the blue sky; why then is it necessary to limit this symbolism to a thread and not extend it to the whole garment? From the standpoint of "commonsense Halakhah," Korah was right. A beautiful *tekhelet* robe will have a greater impact upon the individual than a single thread!

I agree with the preamble of this theory, but only with the preamble. There are indeed two parallel religious orders in Judaism, the objective and the subjective. Judaism consists of both divine discipline (as contained in the *Shulhan Arukh*) and the great romance between man and God, between finitude and infinity (as elaborated in the Song of Songs). Deed and experience are inseparably united.

The deed without experience is an incomplete act, an imperfect gesture. We know that this is correct from the viewpoint of strict halakhic thinking because certain *mitzvot* consist in experience. I am not referring to the mitzvah of love of God or the mitzvah of love of man; I am referring to ritual *mitzvot*. For instance, *keri'at Shema* is strictly identified with the recital of a certain fixed and standardized text; however, the *kiyyum ha-mitzvah,* the realization of the mitzvah, is the inner experience. The same is true of *avodah she-balev*, prayer; of *avelut*, mourning; and of *simhat yom tov*, festival rejoicing. Notwithstanding the halakhic requirement for the recital of standardized texts or the observance of external rites, these *mitzvot* are consummated and realized in an experience. In other words, even the formal abstract Halakhah knows of experience as an important part of the religious gesture.

However, the religious experience is not the primary gesture. The point of departure must never be the inner, subjective experience, no matter how redemptive, colorful, and therapeutic it may be, no matter how great its impact upon the total personality of man. The point of departure must always be the objective, external act. The latter does not symbolically express or interpret the experience; the reverse is true: the experience interprets the act. Here lies the mistake of the subjectivist approach.

There are a variety of reasons for the supremacy of the act over the feeling, of the solid religious reality over the emotion.

First, religious emotion—like any other emotion—is changeable, volatile, and transient.

Second, each individual experiences God, man, and the world in a unique fashion. If the religious act had to adjust itself to the inner feelings of man, we would have to invent constantly changing rituals. The appropriate medium of expression today would be obsolete tomorrow. What is good for me does not behoove my next-door neighbor. If the religious experience were the point of departure, and the religious act had to correspond to the experience, there would be a variety of symbolic actions; we could not speak of a monistic service of God. This kind of ever-changing worship is basically idolatrous. According to the Midrash quoted by Rashi (Num. 16:6, s.v. *zot*), Moses told Korah, "The pagans have many laws, many priests, and they cannot assemble for worship in one temple; we, however, have one God, one ark, one Law, one altar, and one high priest." Monistic worship is constant and not exposed to the winds of change.

There is another reason for giving priority to the act over the experience. We can never determine when an experience is religious and not hedonic and mundane. We know of many nonreligious hedonic emotions which possess enormous power; they are hypnotic and, at first glance, redemptive. One may easily confuse the religious drive with the love impulse, the religious ecstatic craving with the aesthetic yearning of the artist. There are common characteristics in both of them—the quest for exaltedness and infinity.

To substitute secular for religious emotions is, again, an idolatrous method. The pagans of old used to indulge in hypnotic, orgiastic ceremonials, mistakenly identifying them with the religious experience. The Torah prohibited idolatrous practices in the ritual and service of God. "Do not inquire about their gods, saying, 'How did these nations serve their gods? I too will follow those practices.' You shall not do so unto the Lord your God" (Deut. 12:30–31). The Torah had in mind the uninhibited, frenzied, hedonic experiences in which the pagans engaged, the rousing of religious awareness by confrontation with the powerful hypnosis of the aesthetic experience. Using the artistic experience in order to pave the way for a religious mood will not succeed. The religious experience is born in a world of its own; it is born within the religious awareness, not under the pressure of physiological carnal drives, not even provoked by spiritual needs of the human personality, such as the need for beauty.

The religious experience—autonomous, free, and original—moves at its own tempo, within its own unique orbit. This kind of independent experience follows the deed instead of preceding it. To pray, and afterwards to engage in a dance or in a song, is fine. However, to dance in order to pray is futile, because it will not lead to prayer. The great romance follows the divine discipline, not the reverse.

Moses said that if one fulfills the mitzvah of *tzitzit*, then a glance at the *tekhelet* thread may perhaps produce in him the experience of infinity. If we proceed from action to experience, then the *tekhelet* color will remind us of the mystery of existence and our link with God. However, if one fails to conform to the halakhic norm, and contrary to the rules of Halakhah avails himself of a commonsense approach, then looking at the *tekhelet* will produce a mundane, hedonic response, not a religious one.

When Korah and his adherents approached Moses with the problem of "a garment that is entirely *tekhelet*," they wanted a commonsense interpretive approach to Halakhah. They simply had no patience to study, to get the proper training and master the unique halakhic methodology. Of course, Moses ultimately won. We still study the Halakhah in light of Moses' esoteric, conceptualizing logic. The *masorah* of method, of halakhic structures and *a priori* constructs, will continue forever.

We read, "Aaron shall burn there incense, every morning when he tends the lamps, he shall burn it; and when Aaron lights the lamps at dusk, he shall burn it" (Ex. 30:7–8). The burning of the incense and the lighting of the lamps are merged by the Torah into one mitzvah. As a matter of fact, there is a separate *kiyyum* of combining, almost simultaneously, the kindling of the candles with the offering of the incense. Lighting the candles signifies understanding, knowledge of Torah, clarity of concepts, depth in halakhic analysis, a clear deed, intelligent performance. The incense represents the hidden and the intimate, the *mysterium magnum* of creation and the *mysterium tremendum* of the Divine Presence in creation and beyond: "The cloud of incense will cover the ark" (Lev. 16:13).

Ketoret, incense, tells us a great story of the human craving for God, the quest and yearning for the *makor*, the beginning of all. *Ketoret* tells a marvelous story of the tragic human waiting for ecstatic unity with the Almighty. The colorful religious experience is represented by the *ketoret*; the clear religious path and intelligent action are represented by the candles of the *menorah*.

The Torah, however, admonishes us that the burning of the incense is to be coordinated with the lighting, the mystery of feeling with the clarity of thinking and acting, the excitement and passion of experience with the serenity and peace of halakhic comprehension and halakhic implementation. Both are necessary: there are parallel orders of experience and deed, of romance and discipline, of feeling and thought. The incense cannot be separated from the lighting of the candles, and the blue threads cannot be separated from the white. The subjective must never be isolated from the objective. Halakhic detail and precision are necessary if one wants to attain a great and colorful religious experience.

❧ *Moses' Death on the Brink of Return*

Anonymous Years

The Korah incident happened right after the initiation of Aaron into the priesthood in the second year following the Exodus. It was right after Korah's downfall that we read the prophecy, "And the Lord said to Aaron, You and your sons, and your father's house with you, shall bear the iniquity of the Sanctuary" (Num. 18:1). Two chapters later we read, "Then came the children of Israel, the whole congregation, into the desert of Zin, in the first month: and the people abode in Kadesh, and Miriam died there, and was buried there" (Num. 20:1). This verse deals with an event which transpired in the fortieth year, after those who had experienced the Exodus died in the wilderness. Rashi says (s.v. *kol*), " 'The entire congregation' means the congregation in its integrity, for those who were to die in the wilderness [in consequence of their sin] had already died, but these were separated to live."

How strange! The Torah records only two and half years of the Israelites' sojourn in the desert; thirty-eight years in the middle remain anonymous. We have no record of the events that transpired. What did they do? What did they say? What did Moses do during those long, dreary years? Everything is enigmatic, mysterious, frightening.

How tersely and sadly Moses later summarizes the thirty-eight-year sojourn in the wilderness. The sentences are saturated with grief:

> And you returned and wept before the Lord; but the Lord would not hearken to your voice, nor give ear to you. So you abode in Kadesh many days. . . . Then we turned, and took our journey into the wilderness by way of the Red Sea, as the Lord spoke to me, and circled the hill country of Seir many days. . . . And the days in which we came from Kadesh-Barnea, until we crossed the brook Zered, were thirty-eight years, until all the generation of the men of war had perished from the camp, as the Lord had sworn concerning them (Deut. 1:45–2:1, 2:14).

In short, the empty space between Kadesh-Barnea and the resumption of the march to the Promised Land was an era of *hester panim*, the hiding of God's face, and of complete alienation of the people from God. No prayer was accepted, no communication from God reached man; the heavens were insensitive, the world mute, and God very far.

Interesting is that the Torah fills the gap between the second year (chap. 18) and the fortieth year (chap. 20) by narrating the laws of the *parah adumah*, the red heifer (chap. 19). Logically, the section dealing with the *parah adumah* should have appeared in Leviticus, either in the context of the initiation of the Tabernacle service—since, according to our tradition, a red heifer was offered on the eighth day of the preparatory service—or in the context of the laws of purity and impurity. Yet the Torah chose to deal with *tum'at met*, the impurity arising from contact with a dead body (from which one is purified by the *parah adumah*), separately from all other forms of impurity.

Why place it here, in the gap between the second and fortieth years?

The laws of *tum'at met* are the symbol of the thirty-eight years. *Tum'at met* results from the tragic experience of a person who suddenly is forced to realize that his existence is a mockery, that death denies the very worth of human existence. The *tum'ah* is the expression of human anxiety, terror, and helplessness. It represents the human situation, the tragic and absurd human destiny.

Generally, all that is required to remove one's impurity—for example, the impurity that results from contact with the carcass of a dead animal—is *tevillah*, immersion in a *mikveh* or the "living water" of a spring, river, or ocean. But the *tamei met* must be sprinkled with *mei hattat* (spring water mixed with ashes of the red heifer); *tevillah* alone does not suffice. The *tamei met* cannot sprinkle the water upon himself; another person must do it. "And the *tahor*, the clean person, shall sprinkle upon the unclean" (Num. 19:19). "The clean person" who will free the unclean from the bondage of defilement is the Almighty, as the prophet says, "Then I will sprinkle water upon you, and you shall be clean" (Ez. 36:25). Only He will heal man from the threat and terror of nihility; only He will elucidate to us the awesome mystery of death.

How beautifully did *Hazal* portray this dark and dreary night of loneliness when even Moses lost contact with the Almighty. It was a silent, bleak period. The Midrash tells us that "Every Tish'ah be-Av they used to dig graves and spend the night there. On the morrow a voice announced, 'Living separate themselves from the dead' " (Lam. Rabbah, *Petihta* 33). Every Tish'ah be-Av many were ready to die in their graves. Life was not different from death. A life without hope, without anticipation, without a future, is death. No one dreamt, no one prayed for fulfillment; everybody knew what the future held in store for him—a grave on some Tish'ah be-Av. People did not understand God's ways; they were perplexed and frightened. Their whole existence was irrational and absurd. Everyone dug his own grave and lay down in the ditch waiting for the end.

This is one of the most enigmatic, paradoxical eras in history, a period dedicated to death and annihilation. It was a mute time. Man was completely separated from God. Not even the greatest of all men could communicate with Him. The whole community waited for the Almighty's intervention and His redeeming grace, for Him to sprinkle the cleansing waters upon them, for help that comes from somewhere else.

Isn't the section of *parah adumah* the bridge which spans the mysterious river flowing into nowhere, into nihility and oblivion? Isn't this the great and frightening *hukkat ha-Torah* (Num. 19:2), the mystery of "This is the Torah: when a man dies in a tent" (Num. 19:14), the mystery of *haza'ah*? Frightened man cannot free himself from the terror of death. He must look to the *tahor* to help him.

The Torah concludes its narration of the events of the second year by elaborating the laws of priestly gifts and levite tithes (Num. 18), announcing *ipso facto* that no matter how long the delay, the Promised Land will finally be theirs. Suddenly the Torah interrupts the dialogue with Aaron and Moses and bids them farewell; we will resume the conversation, the Almighty said, thirty-eight years from now. Now a period of anonymity and *hester panim*, a period of irrationality and antinomic existence, is about to commence; this period will be known as that of *hukkat ha-Torah*, the mysterious, unintelligible ordinance, when man surrenders his rationality and suspends his judgment to the Almighty. Only at the end of that period, when the congregation stops digging graves, will the dialogue pick up again.

How can one live in such times? The answer is: by faith. The *parashah* of *Zot hukkat ha-Torah*, of defilement by death and purification by the red heifer, is the *parashah* of faith: we believe that finally the "clean person" will sprinkle upon the "unclean person." Is there a more dramatic introduction to the story of the thirty-eight-year period of *hester panim* than the *parah adumah*, with its destiny-charged words, "This is the law (*hukkah*) ordained by the Almighty"? Why is *parah adumah* called a *hukkah*? What is incomprehensible about it is not the ceremonial of the red heifer, but rather the need for special cleansing. Unintelligible is the tragic destiny of man, which necessitates the ceremonial of the *parah*, the ordination (not only halakhic but metaphysical) that "when a man dies in a tent, all that comes into the tent and all that is in the tent shall be unclean for seven days."

When man—successful and creative, a home builder, planner, and architect, an accumulator of wealth—comes face-to-face with death, everything disappears. Death is a traumatic, defiling, and denigrating experience for all. "This is the Torah: when a man dies in a tent" is the proper motto for the untold story of the thirty-eight-year sojourn.

The Enigma and Tragedy of Moses' Death

If death per se is a nauseating, grisly experience which perplexes man, the death of an individual for the sake of atoning for someone else is the most unintelligible experience. Why did Moses die? After all, he was chosen as the redeemer, and he sacrificed his private life for the people. He was the one who received the Torah, the content of which concerned the life of the people not in the desert but in the Promised Land. Why did he not live to see the land he was so eager to see? "And I besought the Lord at that time, saying, O Lord God, You have begun to show Your servant Your greatness and Your mighty hand . . . I pray of You, let me go over, and see the good land that is beyond the Jordan, that goodly mountain region and the Lebanon" (Deut. 3:23–25). And yet, not only was his prayer not accepted; he was even enjoined from praying: "And God was incensed against me . . . and He said to me: 'Enough! Speak no more with Me about this matter' " (Deut. 3:26). Many theories have been advanced by our commentators concerning Moses' death in the desert, but none of the answers satisfies. The Torah uses unequivocal language. It is humanly impossible to grasp the rationality of Moses' death. Death in general, and Moses' death in particular, belongs to the realm of *Zot hukkat ha-Torah*.

Let me elaborate on the enigmatic and tragic aspect of this story. No matter what was the reason for Moses' death, one basic truth stands out: Moses suffered on account of the Children of Israel. The Torah emphasizes this verity a few times: "The Lord was angry with me *because of you*" (Deut. 1:37); "And God was incensed against me *on your account*" (Deut. 3:26). The psalmist states: "And they provoked Him at the waters of Meribah, and Moses suffered *on their account*" (Ps. 106:32). Yet in what regard were the people responsible for Moses' sin? If the sin consisted in hitting the rock instead of addressing words to it, Moses himself was responsible for his deed. The same question applies to the other theories concerning the nature of Moses' guilt.

It was not the fault of the Jewish people that Moses made a mistake. But had the people possessed a sensitivity and love for Moses similar to the love that Moses felt for them, they would have torn the decree into shreds. It was their fault. This is one answer to our question. When he was told that he would not enter the Land of Israel, Moses pleaded for forgiveness. Had the people joined him in prayer, the Holy One would have been forced to respond. But they did not join. Thus we read in *Parashat Va-ethannan* that with tears in his eyes Moses tells them, "*Va-ethannan*" (Deut. 3:23): I prayed alone. It was not *va-nithannan*, we prayed. I was a lonely, solitary prayerful person; I prayed, no one else joined in with me. But God became angry and did not listen to me *lema'ankhem*, because of you.

Yet there is another reason as well. I believe that in studying the chapters dealing with the last months of Moses' life we are confronted with the most touching tragedy—the tragedy of the teacher who is too great for his disciples, the tragedy of the master who is too exalted for the generation. The disciples were not worthy of being Moses' representatives. He had boundless knowledge, enormous depth and sweep, and unqualified morality and saintliness—but his students did not understand him. His singularity caused alienation.

Of course, Joshua, Eleazar, and Phinehas received the Torah from Moses; they carried on Moses' tradition and reflected his glory and majesty. Our Rabbis taught that "Moses' countenance was like the sun"—it radiated its own light; "Joshua's countenance was like the moon"—it reflected light (*Bava Batra* 75a). However, Moses was the teacher par excellence of the entire generation which he delivered from bondage, and particularly of the generation which grew up in the desert under his supervision and tutelage. Why did not the whole nation behave with dignity, humility, discipline, and perseverance in times of distress? Why did they not act in Shittim with firmness and with heroic resistance and determination vis-à-vis temptation and desire, when the lascivious and beautiful daughters of Moab enticed the people (Num. 25)?

When the people made the Golden Calf, Moses argued, "Why should Your wrath be incensed against Your people, whom You took out of Egypt?" (Ex. 32:11). What do You expect them to do, he said. Their background is pagan; they have not been reeducated and retrained in practicing the morality of Abraham, Isaac, and Jacob. It takes time, Moses argued, to reform and rehabilitate a people, to teach them new morals and virtues. It was indeed a sound and solid defense. The generation of those who left Egypt could not be considered the disciples of Moses.

However, in Shittim another generation sinned, the generation of those who *were* brought up by Moses. Just a short time earlier, in the Wilderness of Zin, they had complained to Moses in the same language their fathers had used forty years before: "And why have you made us come up out of Egypt, to bring us in unto this evil place?" (Num. 20:5). Why should Moses' disciples speak the language of liberated slaves who had just parted from the fleshpots? That is why, when they sinned with the daughters of Moab in Shittim, Moses broke down and cried (Num. 25:6 and Ex. Rabbah 33:5). These people were not the students for whom Moses had hoped. Why should the greatest of all teachers fail in his central mission?

Moses did not fail! No! Providence ordained it. Moses was too great for his generation. He rose high above them. His vision was too penetrating, his depth superhuman, his sweep too high. They could not follow him; they failed to understand him. Had they understood and appreciated him, nothing of that sort would have happened, and Moses would have been admitted to the Promised Land. The people's guilt consisted in their not opening up to Moses' influence, in resisting his redemptive and cathartic power, in not being willing to become his disciples. Of course, Moses suffered the consequences. The Halakhah states, "If the student was sentenced to be exiled to a city of refuge, his teacher goes with him into exile" (*Makkot* 10a). The Israelites sinned because they closed their minds and hearts to Moses' teaching and to the richness of his personality. Moses was found guilty—and he was punished.

Again we are confronted with "This is the Torah: when a man dies in a tent," the unintelligibility of the death of a person who did not sin, the mystery of the death of a human being who deserved to live forever. This time the person was the greatest of all men, the man par excellence!

A Tragic Change in our Historical Destiny

Moses' failure to cross the Jordan complicated matters and caused a tragic change in our historical destiny. Had Moses entered the land, the whole history of our people would have taken another turn. It would have been less tragic, less sad, and less mysterious, but at the same time less heroic—and consequently less great.

If *Benei Yisrael* had proven themselves worthy of communing with Moses, of being his disciples, if they had displayed the intellectual and emotional capacity to receive and absorb

Torat Mosheh, then Moses would have entered and conquered the Promised Land, and he would have been anointed as the King Messiah. Jewish history would have found its realization and fulfillment immediately upon entering the land.

There was no reason to deny the messianic role to Moses; he was the greatest of all men. His personality as *adon ha-nevi'im*, the master of prophets, is far superior to that of the King Messiah. Maimonides writes that the Messiah's prophetic capacity will be "close to that of Moses" (*Hilkhot Teshuvah* 9:2); however, Moses will nevertheless retain his superiority. If so, the question arises, why did the Almighty not ordain Moses as the King Messiah? No one else will ever be as qualified as Moses. Had Moses entered and hallowed the land, the *kedushah* would have been eternal; the Babylonian legions could never have annulled it.

The answer is obvious. The messianic era would have commenced if the entire generation, the entire nation, had accepted Moses' message fully. If his teachings had made a genuine impact upon his contemporaries, if these people had indeed become his disciples, if they had treated him with reverence and love the way the *talmid* is supposed to treat his *rebbi*, then Moses would have been ordained as the Messiah.

Unfortunately, they did not rise to the great and singular occasion. *Torat Mosheh* was the possession of a few; the crowd acted like liberated bondmen who could not forget the pots of flesh. After the passage of forty years, the opportunity was missed. The era of the Messiah was postponed for a long period of time; the distance between Moses' redemption and the Messiah's redemption grew almost *ad infinitum*. Moses had to die in the sandhills of Moab. His teachings were entrusted to Joshua, to the people, to countless future generations. Only when the entire congregation has committed itself to this teaching, when Moses is accepted as the master, and when we all demonstrate our capability and readiness to become inquisitive disciples of our master and teacher, only then will the hour of redemption strike. In the interim we must travel a tortuous, long road toward a far destination. Moses did not cross the Jordan; he did not receive the crown of the Messiah. The congregation of Israel was assigned the task of waiting for the Messiah, who could have led us across the Jordan into the Promised Land 3,500 years ago.

The great mystery of death burgeons. Moses died because his contemporaries did not recognize his greatness and moral perfection. Because of his untimely death, Jewish history became longer, more complex, unintelligible and tragic. Moses and the King Messiah, who were supposed to join, separated and turned into two identities, and the Jew learned how to believe and to wait. "This is the Torah: when a man dies in a tent . . ."

"To Judge the Mount of Esau"

The sequence of events as narrated in *Parashat Hukkat* is as follows: The Torah tells us about Miriam, the prophetess of redemption, the little girl who watched the floating ark, the girl with faith and hope who died in the Wilderness of Zin (Num. 20:1). Then the Torah narrates the story of the Waters of Meribah, and we read of Moses' error and the divine oath that neither he nor Aaron would bring the assembly into the Promised Land (20:2–13). It would have been quite understandable if the Torah had told us immediately about Aaron's death (20:22–29); the continuity would have been preserved. Instead the Torah relates another event, namely, the refusal of the king of Edom to lct the Israelites cross his country and the fact that the Israelites were turned away from him (20:14–21).

When Sihon and Og refused to cooperate, Moses declared war and crushed them. Yet Edom was not touched. Once the king categorically declined their request, they changed their route and they compassed Mount Se'ir many days until the people felt exhausted and discouraged because of the steady circling around the land of Edom. Why were they very tolerant toward Edom and very firm vis-à-vis more powerful kingdoms? Of course, we find the answer in Deuteronomy:

> And command the people saying: You are to pass through the boundary of your brethren the children of Esau who abide in Se'ir, and they shall be afraid of you. Take good heed unto yourselves therefore; contend not with them, for I will not give you of their land, not so much as a foot's breadth, because I have given Mount Se'ir unto Esau as a possession (Deut. 2:4–5).

Will the Children of Israel never conquer Mount Se'ir? We are told by the prophet that when the Messiah arrives, "the saviors shall ascend from Mount Zion to judge the Mount of Esau; and the kingdom shall be the Lord's" (Ob. 1:21). However, only then will it happen—not prior to the appearance of the Messiah. Edom is the symbol of the hostility displayed by many toward the Jew; Edom is the antagonist who engaged Jacob in battle in a bleak, dark night; Edom is the perennial opposition the Jew encounters every time he quests for freedom and self-expression; Edom is the mysterious fiend making the life of the Jew difficult. Yes, once Moses was instructed by God to die in the desert, once Moses lost the majestic messianic crown, Edom's territory became unapproachable to the Jew. Israel was enjoined from invading Mount Se'ir. They may conquer any country, but not Mount Se'ir, as Edom-Amalek will exist as long as the Messiah is absent and the vision not fulfilled.

The Almighty told Moses, "You shall not bring this congregation into the land which I have given them" (Num. 20:12). The messianic era became a distant hope thousands of years away; and during this sad interim period Edom is the ruler and king. Had the Jews acted differently at the Waters of Meribah, Moses would have risen to messianic kingship and Edom would have been conquered and destroyed. That is why the Torah narrates the story of Edom's refusal and Israel's obedience to Edom. For at the Waters of Meribah Moses lost the crown of messianic kingship.

Moses' and David's Dreams Unfulfilled

Consider the introductory remark of the author of the Book of Samuel to David's request to build a House of God:

> When the king dwelt in his house and the Lord had given him rest from all his enemies, the king said to Nathan the Prophet, "I am living in a house of cedar, while the Ark of God dwells within the curtain" (II Sam. 7:1–2).

David had reached the stage where he was entitled to be satisfied and happy. He had accomplished a great deal. He had built a house of cedar—and cedar was the strongest material at that time. David was powerful; everybody feared him, and he was respected and loved as well as feared. Should he not have described himself as a man who was happy and safe, one satisfied with himself, not haunted by fear or bad dreams? He had reached the pinnacle of success. Is this not a time to say: "The Lord is my shepherd, I shall not want; He makes me to lie down in green pastures, He leads me beside the still waters; He restores my soul" (Ps. 23:1–3)?

Instead, he said, I live alone in a house of cedar, but the Ark of God has not moved in with me; it remains within the curtains of the Tabernacle. David understood that no matter of what material a house is built, no matter how beautiful the design, a person cannot find a home unless God is with him. He was living in a house of cedar; however, God was not present there. If man's home progresses from an ordinary nomad tent to a luxurious house of cedar, then the home of God must move with him.

Let us listen to Nathan's response:

> Thus says the Lord of Hosts: I took you from the pasture, from following the flock, to be ruler over My people, over

Israel. And I was with you wherever you went, and have cut off all your enemies before you, and have given you a great name, like the name of the great men that are on the earth. Moreover, I have established a place for My people Israel, and planted them, that they may dwell in a place of their own and be troubled no more. Evil men shall not oppress them any more as in the past, since the time that I commanded judges to be over My people Israel. I have given you rest from all your enemies, and the Lord tells you that He will make you a house (II Sam. 7:8–11).

After such an introduction, we surely expect approval. Instead, Nathan continues:

And when the days are fulfilled, and you shall sleep with your fathers, I will set up your seed after you, one of your issue, and I will establish his kingdom. He shall build a house for My name and I will establish his royal throne forever (II Sam. 7:12–13).

There is no explanation here, only a cryptic message. We are not even told explicitly the name of the person who will build the Temple. Puzzling too is the verse "According to all these words, and according to all this vision, so did Nathan speak to David" (II Sam. 7:17). Of what great vision had the prophet spoken? Nathan had simply delivered the message that David would not build the Temple but that his seed would. It is only in Chronicles that the explanation is spelled out.

The word of the Lord came to me saying, "You have shed much blood and have made great wars; you shall not build a house for My name, because you have shed much blood upon the earth in My sight. But you will have a son who shall be a man of rest, for I will give him rest from all his enemies; his name will be Solomon, *Shelomo*, and I will confer peace, *shalom*, and quiet on Israel in his days. He shall build a house for My name . . ." (I Chr. 22:8–10).

To understand Nathan's message in the Book of Samuel, we must appreciate that the commandment to build the Temple was closely associated with the state of the kingdom at all levels—political, economic, and military. When the Jews were about to cross the Jordan and enter the Land of Israel, they were told to do three things: appoint a king, defeat Amalek, and build a Temple. Only after having defeated all his enemies and having provided the land with security, safety, and long-lasting peace may the king be called upon to construct the Sanctuary.

The Torah says, "But when you cross the Jordan and dwell in the land which the Lord your God gave to you, to inherit, and He grants you rest from all your enemies about you, so that you shall dwell in safety—then it shall come to pass, that the place which the Lord your God shall choose to cause His name to dwell there, there you shall bring all that I command you" (Deut. 12:10–11). To be frank, we have never been in a position of resting from all our enemies. We could never boast such a victory. We could never say that all the promises came true and that we may dismiss war, persecution, and injustice from our minds. (Of course, in Solomon's time, peace prevailed; but the years were few in number, and already during Solomon's life the kingdom began to fall apart.)

The vision of "And He gives you rest from all your enemies" is still a promise which will be fulfilled, but not before the Messiah has come. Only then will the great universal peace prevail forever, only then will the words of Isaiah be fulfilled: "They shall not hurt nor destroy in all My holy mountain: for the earth shall be full of the knowledge of the Lord, as the waters cover the sea" (Is. 11:9). Only then will we see the realization of the prophecy:

> And I will make them one nation in the land upon the mountains of Israel: and one king shall be king over them all, and they shall be no more two nations. Nor shall they defile themselves any more. . . . And David My servant shall be king over them; and they all shall have one shepherd. They shall also follow My judgments and observe My statutes and do them (Ez. 37:22–24).

Only then will the commandment of building the Temple become binding. Of course, I mean not a temporary Temple, but the ultimate one that will last forever.

The individual who will build this Temple is not the historical David, but his descendant and reincarnation, the Messiah. Indeed, the phrase "And I will set up your seed after you" does not necessarily refer to one's son. When the same phrase is used in God's promise to Abraham, "I will establish My covenant between Me and you and your seed after you" (Gen. 17:7), it means Abraham's descendants. When we speak of David as Messiah, we speak of the personification of a great idea.

King David could not build the Temple for the same reason that Moses could not cross into the Land of Israel. Had Moses crossed the border, the Land of Israel never could have been taken away from the Jewish people. And since Providence planned differently, Moses died on the far shore of the Jordan. Had David built a Temple, no power in the world could have destroyed it. But Providence has decreed differently for our people. A Sanctuary built by David would have had to usher in an era of peace and salvation for all, forever. In the time of King David, the world was not ready for the King Messiah.

From the viewpoint of human reason, the redemption in Egypt should have been the only one in Jewish history. The messianic era should have commenced with the Exodus. God said, "I will take you to Me for a people . . . and I will bring you into the land" (Ex. 6:7); why, then, did those who left Egypt die in the desert and never enter the Land of Israel? Why were the

Jews exiled from their land the first time? Why the second time? Why all the suffering in antiquity, the Middle Ages, and particularly in our time—the Holocaust? Are not the words of *zot hukkat ha-Torah* applicable to our total historical experience? Our whole existence is a mystery, an enigma!

The entire Haggadah is permeated with the question of why we are still slaves, not to Pharaoh but to others. Is not the phrase *hashata avdei*, "This year we are slaves," self-contradictory? Declaring ourselves to be slaves contradicts the very sanctity of the "Night of Watching," the night of the Exodus.

Yet we believe that at some point in time all contradictions will be resolved and the Almighty will purge the historical order of contradictions and antithetic elements. At present the redemption from Egypt is still classified under *zot hukkat ha-Torah*. It will be explained through the intervention of God, "the clean person shall sprinkle upon the unclean." The Exodus will finally be completely realized; the eschatological era will begin; only then will the redemption from Egypt be endowed with its final meaning.

🐝 Index of Biblical and Rabbinic Sources

❧ Index of Topics and Names